T0263159

Obesity in Critically Ill Patients

Guest Editor

LINDA HARRINGTON, PhD, RN, CNS, CPHQ

CRITICAL CARE NURSING CLINICS OF NORTH AMERICA

www.ccnursing.theclinics.com

Consulting Editor
JANET FOSTER, PhD, RN, CNS

September 2009 • Volume 21 • Number 3

SAUNDERS an imprint of ELSEVIER, Inc.

W.B. SAUNDERS COMPANY
A Division of Elsevier Inc.

Elsevier Inc., 1600 John F. Kennedy Blvd., Suite 1800, Philadelphia, PA 19103-2899

http://www.theclinics.com

CRITICAL CARE NURSING CLINICS OF NORTH AMERICA Volume 21, Number 3
September 2009 ISSN 0899-5885, ISBN-13: 978-1-4377-1206-3, ISBN-10: 1-4377-1206-1

Editor: Katie Hartner
Developmental Editor: Donald Mumford

Critical Care Nursing Clinics of North America (ISSN 0899-5885) is published quarterly by Elsevier Inc., 360 Park Avenue South, New York, NY 10010-1710. Months of issue are March, June, September, and December. Business and Editorial Offices: 1600 John F. Kennedy Blvd., Suite 1800, Philadelphia, PA 19103-2899. Periodicals postage paid at New York, NY and additional mailing offices. Subscription prices are $130.00 per year for US individuals, $233.00 per year for US institutions, $68.00 per year for US students and residents, $167.00 per year for Canadian individuals, $292.00 per year for Canadian institutions, $191.00 per year for international individuals, $292.00 per year for international institutions and $99.00 per year for Canadian and foreign students/residents. To receive student/resident rate, orders must be accompanied by name of affiliated institution, data of term, and the *signature* of program/residency coordinator on institution letterhead. Orders will be billed at individual rate until proof of status is received. Foreign air speed delivery is included in all *Clinics* subscription prices. All prices are subject to change without notice. **POSTMASTER:** Send address changes to *Critical Care Nursing Clinics of North America*, Elsevier Health Sciences Division, Subscription Customer Service, 3251 Riverport Lane, Maryland Heights, MO 63043. **Customer Service: 1-800-654-2452 (US and Canada); 314-447-8871 (outside US and Canada). Fax: 314-447-8029. E-mail: JournalsCustomerService-usa@elsevier.com (for print support) and JournalsOnlineSupport-usa@elsevier.com (for online support).**

Reprints. For copies of 100 or more of articles in this publication, please contact the Commercial Reprints Department, Elsevier Inc., 360 Park Avenue South, New York, New York, 10010-1710; Tel.: (212) 633-3813, Fax: (212) 462-1935, and E-mail: reprints@elsevier.com.

Critical Care Nursing Clinics of North America is covered in *MEDLINE/PubMed (Index Medicus)*, *International Nursing Index*, *Nursing Citation Index*, *Cumulative Index to Nursing and Allied Health Literature*, and *RNdex Top 100*.

Printed and bound by CPI Group (UK) Ltd, Croydon, CR0 4YY

Transferred to Digital Print 2011

Contributors

CONSULTING EDITOR

JANET FOSTER, PhD, RN, CNS
Associate Professor, College of Nursing, Texas Women's University, Houston, Texas

GUEST EDITOR

LINDA HARRINGTON, PhD, RN, CNS, CPHQ
Vice President for Advancing Nursing Practice, Baylor Health Care System, Dallas, Texas

AUTHORS

SONIA M. ASTLE, RN, MS, CCRN, CCNS
Clinical Nurse Specialist, Department of Critical Care, Inova Fairfax Hospital, Falls Church, Virginia

MICHELE BEDNARZYK, MN, FNP, BC
Senior Instructor, Brooks College of Health, School of Nursing, University North Florida, Jacksonville, Florida; Certified Family Nurse Practitioner, Volunteers in Medicine-Jacksonville, Jacksonville, Florida

KATHLEEN FEDYSZEN, RN, BSN
Presbyterian Hospital of Plano, Plano, Texas

JANET KLOOS, RN, PhD, CNS, CCRN
Clinical Nurse Specialist, University Hospitals, Case Medical Center, Cleveland, Ohio

V. TERECEITA LAIDLOW, MS, RN, CCRN
Health Initiatives Specialist/Advanced Practice Nurse, Department of Nursing Administration, Sinai Hospital of Baltimore, Baltimore, Maryland

BARBARA LEEPER, MN, RN, CNS, CCRN, FAHA
Clinical Nurse Specialist, Cardiovascular Services, Baylor University Medical Center, Dallas, Texas

JEANNE REDLIN LOWE, PhD(C), RN, CWCN
Clinical Associate Faculty, School of Nursing, Biobehavioral Nursing and Health Systems, University of Washington, Seattle, Washington

BEVERLY MALONEY, RN, MSN, APRN, CCRN
Clinical Nurse Specialist Critical Care, Fairview Hospital CCHS, Cleveland, Ohio

MARGARET McATEE, MN, RN
Critical Care Educator, Baylor All Saints Medical Center, Fort Worth, Texas

WENDY C. PEAVY, MSN, RN, CCRN-CSC, ACNS-BC
Clinical Nurse Specialist, Critical Care Services, Baylor Medical Center at Irving, Irving, Texas

REBECCA J. PERSONETT, PhD
Professor of Nursing, Brookhaven Community College, Dallas, Texas

SUSAN SMITH, MS, RN, CNS
ICU Clinical Nurse Specialist, Texas Health Presbyterian Hospital Plano, Plano, Texas

DEBRA SIELA, PhD, RN, CCNS, ACNS-BC, CCRN, CNE, RRT
Assistant Professor of Nursing, Ball State University, School of Nursing, Muncie, Indiana; ICU Clinical Nurse Specialist, Ball Memorial Hospital, Muncie, Indiana

SHERRY N. VANHOY, MSN, RN, ACNS-BC, CEN
Advanced Practice Nurse, Department of Emergency Medicine, Sinai Hospital of Baltimore, Baltimore, Maryland

MARK WELLIVER, DNP, CRNA, ARNP
Associate Professor of Professional Practice, School of Nurse Anesthesia, Harris College of Nursing and Health Sciences, Texas Christian University, Forth Worth, Texas

CHRIS WINKELMAN, RN, PhD, CCRN, ACNP
Assistant Professor, Frances Payne Bolton School of Nursing, Case Western Reserve University, Cleveland, Ohio

Contents

manage pain effectively for the critically ill obese patient, nurses must have an understanding of how obesity alters a patient's physiologic response to injury and illness. In addition, nurses must be knowledgeable about physiologic pain mechanisms, types and manifestations of pain, differing patterns of drug absorption and distribution, pharmacokinetic properties of analgesic medications, and pain management strategies. This article explores factors affecting pharmacokinetics in obese patients, trends in pain management, and treatment strategies for the obese patient.

Sedation of the obese critical care patient presents unique challenges that include altered respiratory function and a predisposition to respiratory suppression and airway obstruction. Sedative drugs have pronounced effects on obese patients. Knowledge of the anatomic and physiologic changes associated with obesity, airway management, and sedation agents better prepares one to care for these patients safely and effectively.

Caring for obese critically ill patients is not always the same as caring for critically ill patients who are not obese. Fortunately, nurses have many resources available to them to guide them in this process. However, research that specifically addresses the needs of obese critically ill patients is still lacking in many areas and should be considered as potential areas to develop evidence-based practices.

Obesity has become a major health problem in the United States and is well known to be a risk factor for the development of cardiovascular disease. Many clinicians perceive obesity, particularly severe or morbid obesity, to be associated with increased risk for mortality and morbidity following coronary artery bypass graft (CABG) surgery. This article provides a review of the literature related to mortality and morbidity, including the impact of diabetes, risk for acute respiratory failure, and sternal wound infection associated with obese patients undergoing CABG surgery. Implications for nursing practice are addressed with recommendations for practice in this patient population.

Recently, the impact of obesity on the outcomes of trauma patients has been the focus of several investigations. There have been several studies addressing the impact of obesity on trauma patients. These studies have explicated the impact of obesity on negative outcomes of trauma patients. Several studies have identified a relationship between obesity and injury pattern, increased complications in outcomes related to surgical procedures, and increase mortality and morbidity rates in obese trauma patients. However, the literature in nursing management in this patient population is virtually nonexistent and vague. The purpose of this article is to delineate the nursing implications of obesity in trauma patients and to provide guidelines for care of obese trauma patients.

In America today, more than one third of adults are obese. Increasingly, obese patients are admitted to critical care units. Critical care nurses must have additional knowledge and skills to identify health risks to obese patients and implement interventions to prevent untoward problems. Critical care nurses are also at risk when taking care of obese patients. The purpose of this article is to identify risks to both patients and nurses and to provide recommendations to address those risks.

Obese patients in the ICU present unique challenges to the health care team and specific challenges to nurses. This article reviews the science and art of resource use for obese patients in the ICU. Staff nurses and advanced practice nurses can make important contributions in evaluating optimal resource use and improving outcomes in this population of vulnerable patients.

FORTHCOMING ISSUES

December 2009

Neuroscience Nursing
Anne W. Alexandrov, PhD, RN, CCRN,
FAAN, *Guest Editor*

March 2010

Diagnostic Testing
Stephen Krau, PhD, RN, CNE, CT
Guest Editor

June 2010

Liver Failure
Sarah Saxer, PharmD, and
Dinesh Yogaratnam, PharmD, BCPS
Guest Editors

RECENT ISSUES

June 2009

The High-Risk Neonate: Part II
M. Terese Verklan, PhD, CCNS, RNC
Guest Editor

March 2009

The High-Risk Neonate: Part I
M. Terese Verklan, PhD, CCNS, RNC,
Guest Editor

December 2008

**Innovative Practice Models for Acute
and Critical Care**
Maria R. Shirey, PhDc, MS, MBA, RN,
NEA-BC, FACHE, *Guest Editor*

THE CLINICS ARE NOW AVAILABLE ONLINE!

Access your subscription at:
www.theclinics.com

Preface

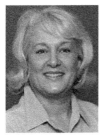

Linda Harrington, PhD, RN, CNS, CPHQ
Guest Editor

This issue of *Critical Care Nursing Clinics* tackles a significant and growing issue in critical care: obesity. Obese patients pose unique challenges to critical care nurses and the increasing numbers of these patients make this an important area of study.

The articles in this issue delve into the impact of obesity on critically ill adult patients, nursing staff, and hospital resources. Nurses will learn how to alter their approaches to assessment, goal setting, care planning, intervention, and evaluation based on the presence of obesity in their patient population. Staff will also learn measures to prevent injury and provide safe patient care.

From the perspective of body systems, authors explore the unique effects of obesity on the cardiovascular system, the pulmonary system, the skin, and nutrition. Authors also explore the disease burden associated with obesity in patients following cardiovascular surgery and trauma. The articles on pain and sedation contain important information for all nurses caring for critically ill patients.

The authors have done an excellent job in gleaning key findings from the current literature. It is evident, however, that more research is needed in this area. This is especially true with regard to the morbidly obese patient.

It is expected that readers will come away from this issue of *Critical Care Nursing Clinics* with a deeper appreciation of the impact of obesity in the critical care setting. Nurses will gain a better understanding of current evidence-based practices for use when intervening in this patient population. It is hoped that some nurses will be inspired to further study the area of critically ill obese patients to generate new knowledge and move us forward.

Linda Harrington, PhD, RN, CNS, CPHQ
Vice President for Advancing Nursing Practice
Baylor Health Care System
Office of the CNO, Suite 600
Bryan Tower, Dallas, TX 75201, USA

E-mail address:
Linda.harrington@gmail.com

Crit Care Nurs Clin N Am 21 (2009) ix
doi:10.1016/j.ccell.2009.07.014
0899-5885/09/$ – see front matter © 2009 Elsevier Inc. All rights reserved.

ccnursing.theclinics.com

Cardiovascular Effects of Obesity: Implications for Critical Care

Wendy C. Peavy, MSN, RN, CCRN-CSC, ACNS-BC

KEYWORDS

- Obesity • Cardiovascular system • Central obesity
- Heart disease • Metabolic syndrome

The literature describes obesity as an epidemic.[1,2] In actuality, obesity has reached pandemic proportions and should be considered a global health crisis. According to the World Health Organization (WHO), globally there are more than 1.6 billion overweight adults, of whom 400 million meet criteria for obesity.[2] Even more disturbing is that this crisis is not restricted to the adult population; it is rapidly impinging upon children. In 2005, the WHO estimated that, worldwide, approximately 20 million children under the age of 5 years were overweight.[2]

Obesity is nondiscriminate and affects all races, ethnicities, genders, and age groups. Although there are disparities in the prevalence of obesity among these groups, they all are affected. The last 30 years has seen a marked increase in the prevalence of obesity: rates for adults have doubled, and rates for children have tripled.[1,2] More recent data released from the Centers for Disease Control report no significant change in obesity prevalence between 2003–2004 and 2005–2006 for men or women.[3] Nonetheless, the numbers remain staggering. In 2005–2006, in the United States alone, more than 72 million adults, 34.4% of the adult population, met the criteria for obesity.[1–3]

Obesity can be defined as excessive body fat and occurs when body weight exceeds the ideal weight by 75%.[4,5] The most commonly used measurement of obesity is body mass index (BMI). The mathematical equation used to determine BMI is weight in kilograms divided by height in meters squared. A BMI greater than 25 kg/m² is considered overweight, a BMI greater than 30 kg/m² is considered obese, and a BMI greater than 40 kg/m² is considered morbidly obese. This weight classification system was identified in a 1998 report published by the National Heart, Lung, and Blood Institute of the National Institutes of Health.[2,4,6,7]

Obesity has become such a health concern that several government and health care agencies have devised initiatives to address this crisis. One of these initiatives is The

Critical Care Services, Baylor Medical Center at Irving, 1901 North MacArthur, Irving, TX 75061, USA
E-mail address: wendy.peavy@baylorhealth.edu

Crit Care Nurs Clin N Am 21 (2009) 293–300
doi:10.1016/j.ccell.2009.07.005
0899-5885/09/$ – see front matter © 2009 Elsevier Inc. All rights reserved.

Healthy People 2010 campaign. Its objectives include a reduction in the prevalence of obesity to 15%, half the actual current prevalence.[3] If the problem is to be addressed effectively and efficiently, it is imperative that every effort be made to solicit active participation in these campaigns. Failure to acknowledge the magnitude and complexity of obesity and its implications will result in insurmountable consequences.

The repercussions resulting from obesity on public health and the health care system are almost unfathomable. Obesity is associated with an increased risk of type 2 diabetes, cardiovascular disease, stroke, and certain types of cancer, obstructive sleep apnea, respiratory dysfunction, dyslipidemia, liver and gallbladder disease, and an overall increased risk in mortality and morbidity.[1-17] The cost of obesity-related health care is phenomenal. In 2000, these costs totaled an estimated $117 billion, and that figure is expected to climb if the problem continues to run rampant.[1,9]

To manage this crisis, it no is longer acceptable just to consider the amount of body fat a person possesses. Research has revealed that the distribution of body fat is as significant as the amount of body fat. Central or abdominal adipose tissue has been shown to be metabolically more active than peripherally distributed fat and is associated with more metabolic complications such as dyslipidemia, diabetes mellitus, and a higher incidence of mortality from ischemic heart disease.[4] Central obesity is one of the several characteristics of the condition termed "syndrome X" or "metabolic syndrome" by Reaven in 1988.[7,8,11] Syndrome X is a collection of metabolic deviations that occur concomitantly in the same person, increasing the risk for heart disease and diabetes mellitus.[6-8,11]

A discussion of the effect of obesity on the cardiovascular system is warranted, because obesity has been identified as a strong and independent risk factor for heart failure, ischemic heart disease, and obesity-induced cardiomyopathy.[4,6,9,10,12,15] It is essential that this knowledge be considered during assessment, treatment, and care of the obese patient by critical care nurses.

ALTERATIONS IN CARDIOVASCULAR STRUCTURE

The most notable structural derangement of the cardiovascular system in the obese adult population is the remodeling of the heart, more specifically the ventricles. This remodeling transpires over time through multiple chains of events and is related directly to the degree of obesity, the duration of obesity, and any concomitant disease processes such as hypertension and diabetes.[13] In a postmortem study of 76 individuals who had a BMI greater than 30 kg/m^2, 100% of the individuals had a postmortem diagnosis of cardiomegaly, and 64% received a diagnosis of left ventricular hypertrophy (LVH).[4,14,15] In fact, the evidence revealed a linear relationship between cardiac weight and body weight up to 105 kg, after which the weight of the heart continued to increase but at a slower rate.[4,14,15] There continues to be a lack of consensus regarding the definitive cause of the increased cardiac weight, however. Some researchers attribute this increase to excess epicardial fat, but others attribute the increase to ventricular hypertrophy.[14]

The remodeling process begins with an increase in blood volume and cardiac output. The increased total blood volume is needed to meet the perfusion needs of the additional amount of adipose tissue.[4,6,9,12,15,16] Adipose tissue is no longer referred to as just "fat" it is now considered an endocrine organ that is capable of synthesizing and releasing into the bloodstream peptides and nonpeptide compounds, such as atrial natriuretic peptide and the rennin-substrate angiotensin (which regulate fluid volume), and these substances may play a role in cardiovascular homeostasis.[6]

The increase in intracellular and extracellular volume contributes to an elevation in the stroke volume and ultimately the cardiac output, but there is no compensatory increase in the heart rate. The increased cardiac output eventually leads to ventricular enlargement and hypertrophy of both the left and right ventricles. These physiological changes accompanied by alterations in ventricular function have been designated "obesity-induced cardiomyopathy."[4,5,15]

In response to the increase in the left ventricular filling pressures and volume, the chamber of the heart becomes dilated or enlarged. This dilation eventually leads to increased strain on the walls of the ventricle, increased myocardial mass, and LVH.[5,6,15] Ventricular hypertrophy produced through the aforementioned process is known as "eccentric LVH."

The addition of hypertension to this process (some obese patients that are normotensive) contributes to concentric LVH. Concentric LVH is the thickening of the ventricular walls secondary to increased pressures. More often than not, patients who present with obesity and hypertension present with a combination of eccentric and concentric LVH.[5,6,9,15,17] This remodeling of the heart is usually considered irreversible.

These physiological changes to the left ventricle coupled with stiffening of the ventricle wall contribute to both left ventricular systolic and diastolic dysfunction. This dysfunction compounded by ischemic heart disease ultimately leads to left ventricular failure.[4,12,15] At this point, weight loss will assist only in the minimization of symptoms because the damage is irreversible.

The structural changes to the right ventricle occur as a result of the effects of obesity on the respiratory system as well as the cardiovascular system. Obese people are afflicted with obstructive sleep apnea as well as obesity hypoventilation syndrome.[4] These conditions lead to chronic hypoxia and hypercapnia and ultimately to pulmonary hypertension, both arterial and venous. Pulmonary arterial hypertension is a contributing factor to right ventricular enlargement and hypertrophy and eventually right-sided heart failure.[4]

ALTERATIONS IN CARDIOVASCULAR FUNCTION

Alterations in the cardiovascular function occur most often in the form of left ventricular diastolic dysfunction secondary to both eccentric and concentric LVH. As mentioned earlier, the thickening of the myocardial wall results in decreased compliance. In addition, impairment of ventricular filling leads to an increased left ventricular end diastolic pressure, left ventricular end diastolic volume, and pulmonary edema.[4,6] The stiff ventricle limits the force of contraction necessary to eject the blood from the ventricle, resulting in a decreased ejection fraction. In some cases, the ventricle cannot continue to become hypertrophied once it reaches a certain point. In this scenario the ventricle continues to dilate, the walls cease to hypertrophy, and systolic dysfunction follows.[4]

Several other alterations in cardiovascular function include, but are not limited to, venous insufficiency, elevated blood viscosity, and hemodynamics.[12,15] Venous insufficiency is the result of lymphatic overload and increased intravascular volume secondary to an increase in blood volume. This insufficiency, coupled with a decrease in activity common in obese individuals, can result in a back flow of blood in the leg veins because of venous valvular incompetence.[15] The resultant venous stasis increases an individual's risk of pretibial ulcerations, cellulitis, venous thrombosis, and pulmonary embolism.[15] This condition is further complicated by the increase in blood viscosity.

As previously mentioned, adipose cells have been associated with the secretion of many substances that effect homeostasis. One of these substances is plasminogen activator inhibitor-I (PAI-1) protein. This protein is the chief inhibitor of the fibrinolytic system. Overproduction of PAI-1 may contribute to dysfunction of the fibrinolytic system and result in coagulopathy.[6,12] Leptin, a hormone known to be secreted by fat cells, has been associated with an increase in platelet aggregation,[6,12] increasing even further the risk of venous thrombosis, pulmonary embolism, and coagulopathy.

Manifestations of hemodynamic alterations include an increase in cardiac output, right atrial pressure, right ventricular end diastolic pressure, and pulmonary artery mean and occlusive pressures[6,12] and are a direct result of the effects of increased blood volume present in obese individuals. These alterations contribute to the previously discussed process of the remodeling of the heart ventricles and ultimately to obesity-induced cardiomyopathy. Furthermore, there is a maladaptive neural regulation of the circulation in the presence of excess adipose tissue.[12] The increased hemodynamic load in combination with impairment of neural regulation contributes to oxidative stress, all of which lead to further progression of left ventricular remodeling[12] and eventual heart failure.

IMPLICATIONS FOR NURSING PRACTICE
Assessment

Assessment of the obese patient often is challenging for the critical care nurse, and alterations in the assessment may be necessary. Strategies for performing the most comprehensive and accurate assessment for this patient population are essential. Some of the simplest portions of the assessment, for example, auscultation of heart sounds, can become the most difficult. The excess body fat in the obese patient can make it difficult to assess heart sounds, especially murmurs. Heart sounds often are distant or muffled in the obese patient. Strategies such as turning off the television, closing doors, or minimizing the extraneous noise of equipment may help the critical care nurse in the assessment.[6] Additional strategies include placing the patient in the left lateral position or sitting up at a 45° angle to bring the heart nearer to the chest wall.[6]

When assessing the point of maximal impulse (PMI), it is important for the critical care nurse to note that that it may be misplaced secondary to an enlarged heart or a horizontal shift of the heart. The PMI normally is located in the fourth or fifth intercostal space just medial to the left midclavicular line. In the obese patient, the PMI may be auscultated or palpated closer to the midaxillary line.

In the obese patient the heart must pump an increased blood volume against an increased systemic vascular resistance.[6,16] The increased oxygen demand and energy needs of the obese patient translate into a compensatory tachycardia and hypertension.[6] Hence, obese patients have a higher incidence of tachycardia secondary to the increased workload on the myocardium.[6,16]

When assessing the blood pressure of an obese patient, the critical care nurse must be vigilant in selecting a blood pressure cuff. In the ideal setting, a critically ill patient in the ICU would have an arterial line to monitor the blood pressure, but this is not always the case. Guidelines for cuff size should be followed. Normally, to obtain the most accurate blood pressure measurement, the cuff bladder should be greater than or equal to 80% of the patient's arm circumference, and the width of the cuff should be greater than or equal to 40% of the arm circumference.[6,16] An accurate blood pressure measurement in the critically ill patient is essential in the guidance of treatment.

Assessment of peripheral pulses, especially pedal pulses, may need to be performed by Doppler ultrasound[6] if the patient has severe peripheral vascular disease or extreme edema to the lower extremities. As discussed earlier, obese patients may have marked edema in the lower extremities secondary to venous insufficiency. The presence of edema in the lower extremities makes it difficult to assess peripheral pulses and also makes it difficult to assess for cellulitis and deep vein thrombosis (DVT).

Obesity has been designated as an independent risk factor for the development of venous thromboembolism.[4,6,9,15,16] Increased tissue mass secondary to excess adipose tissue and lower extremity edema may disguise the swelling in patients who develop DVT. The critical care nurse may need to alter the assessment to include a more focused assessment of the lower extremities that includes circulation, pain, and warmth.[6] The use of antiembolism stockings or sequential compression devices in DVT prophylaxis is considered the standard of care. In some patients, their size does not allow the use of properly fitting equipment. In such cases creativity and innovation are essential. One example is wrapping the legs with elastic bandages to produce an equivalent effect.[6] Additional prevention tactics include conducting scheduled range of motion exercises and the use of low molecular weight heparin.[6]

Standard hemodynamic parameters that can be indexed to the individual patient should be measured and recorded whenever possible.[6] Parameters indexed to the individual are more accurate and provide a more precise guideline for monitoring and treatment, especially when titrating medications. As previously mentioned, alterations in hemodynamics include an increase in cardiac output, right atrial pressure, right ventricular end diastolic pressure, and pulmonary artery mean and occlusive pressures.[6,12]

ECG Changes

Changes in the ECG often are the result of alterations in the morphology of the myocardium. Conduction intervals often exhibit an increase in length secondary to the hypertrophied myocardium. These ECG changes include an increased PR interval, QRS complex, and QT interval.[15] Other ECG changes include ST depression, left axis deviation, and low QRS voltage.[15] In addition, obese patients have greater incidence of false-positive criteria for inferior myocardial infarctions, which are thought to be the result of diaphragmatic elevation secondary to excess adipose tissue.[15]

Additional influences on ECG changes in the obese patient include a horizontal shift of the heart, which usually appears as a nonspecific flattening of the T wave in the inferolateral leads,[15] and many other nonspecific changes that may be related to an increased distance of the electrodes from the heart secondary to increased tissue mass.[15] In the absence of known concomitant disease processes, these changes are the often first signs of obesity-induced derangements of the myocardium. Many of these patients are asymptomatic because of their sedentary lifestyles,[15] and an astute critical care nurse may be the first practitioner to associate the ECG changes with the commencement of the cardiac remodeling process and eventual development of obesity-induced cardiomyopathy.

Arrhythmias

Arrhythmias in the obese patient may be the result of structural changes in the heart or other conditions associated with obesity. Arrhythmias are exacerbated by acute and chronic illnesses. Conditions that may lead to cardiac arrhythmias include, but are not limited to, hypoxia, hypercapnia, electrolyte disturbances (often brought on by diuretic therapy), increased circulating catecholamine concentrations, and fatty permeation of the cardiac conduction system.[4,6] Premature ventricular contractions often are seen in patients who have concentric LVH, and the incidence of atrial fibrillation is higher in obese patients secondary to fluid overload and dilation of the atria.[6]

It is vital that the critical care nurse be aware of such information while caring for the obese patient. This knowledge is helpful in determining the cause of arrhythmias and allows the nurse and health care team to make a preemptive strike to prevent arrhythmias. Furthermore, it allows appropriate treatment selections when prevention has been unsuccessful.

Positioning

Positioning is an important consideration when caring for the obese patient. In addition to the advantage of positioning during assessment, positioning is important in the prevention of atelectasis, pulmonary edema, gastric reflux, and aspiration pneumonia.[4,9,16] Obese patients have a decrease in diaphragmatic excursion because of the presence of excess adipose tissue, especially abdominal adipose tissue.[9,18] This reduced excursion increases the risk of atelectasis, particularly in the supine position.[9,18]

Obese patients have increased cardiac filling pressures at rest. The pressures increase further when the patient is supine. The supine position creates an environment conducive to the formation of pulmonary edema in the critically ill obese patient and should be avoided when possible.[4,9,16]

Traditionally, elevating the head of the bed has been the standard of care to prevent atelectasis, pulmonary edema, gastric reflux, and aspiration pneumonia. It has been suggested, however, that obese patients in the critical care setting, once hemodynamically stable, should be placed in the reverse Trendelenburg position at a 45° angle.[9,18] This position maximizes the diaphragmatic excursion of the patient and decreases the risk of complications.

It would be remiss not to mention comfort and skin care when discussing positioning. Obese patients often require special-sized beds (often called "bariatric beds"). These beds are larger, to accommodate the obese patient. Patients can be turned and repositioned more comfortably. Furthermore, the larger bed prevents the patient from being squeezed between the bedrails, which promotes skin breakdown.

It is imperative that critical care nurses be vigilant when providing skin care. Obese patients have multiple skin folds that are prone to moisture and, if not cleaned well, foster bacteria and yeast,[9] making the skin more susceptible to breakdown. Breakdown further complicates the recovery of the obese patient and increases the risk of infections.

Pharmacology

Medication therapy in the obese patient can be complicated. Standard guidelines for medication dosing in obese patients are scarce. Many factors affect medication distribution, including body composition, regional blood flow, and affinity for plasma proteins.[16] These factors are altered in the obese patient, especially the critically ill obese patient, creating the potential for under- or overtreatment.

It has been suggested that total body weight be used when dosing medications, especially in obese patients.[16,19] There always are exceptions to the rule, however. In the case of fentanyl, an analgesic, it has been suggested that a corrected dosing weight be used, because there is not a linear relationship between clearance and total body weight above 70 kg.[16] The corrected dosing weight is known as the "pharmokinetic mass."[16,20]

Another factor affecting medication distribution in obese patients is the classification of the medication. Some medications, such as propofol, fentanyl, and the benzodiazepines, are lipophilic; other medications, such as antimicrobials and the neuromuscular blockers, are hydrophilic. The volume of distribution of these medications is multifactorial, as previously mentioned. The critical care nurse must be aware that in obese patients the increased fat to muscle ratio, or body composition, alters this volume of distribution.[9,16,19]

The increased fat to muscle ratio alters not only medication distribution and clearance but the patient's therapeutic response as well.[9,16,19] Patients in critical care areas should be monitored closely using pain, sedation, and agitation scales. Medications should be titrated accordingly.

There is no single authority or consensus on the dosing of medications in obese patients. Opinions differ as to which weight (total body weight, ideal body weight, pharmokinetic mass, or lean body weight) should be used when dosing medications for the critically ill obese patient.[9] This lack of consensus presents an extraordinary challenge in emergency situations, because the guidelines for advanced cardiac life support (ACLS) medications are weight based.[19] After an extensive review of the literature, Harrington and Leiker[19] reported that there are no consistent guidelines for weight-based dosing of ACLS medications in obese patients.

SUMMARY

Obesity has become a major global health crisis. The condition usually is chronic and rarely exists alone. Its causes are multifactorial and complex. These patients present a challenge to the critical care nurse and to the health care team. It is imperative that a transdisciplinary health team be assembled to care for these patients and that the team is armed with knowledge of the physiological alterations in the structure and function of the cardiovascular system and all other body systems, as well. This knowledge will assist the health care team in promoting safe passage of the patient through the health care system as well as through the patient's life span.

ACKNOWLEDGEMENTS

The author thanks Dr Linda Harrington, PhD, RN, CNS, CHPQ, Scott Williams, MSN-HCSM, RN, NE-BC, RN-BCCV, and Jame Restau, MSN, RN, ACNS-BC, OCN for their assistance with this article.

REFERENCES

1. Centers for Disease Control and Prevention. Obesity: halting the epidemic by making health easier, 2009. Available at: www.cdc.gov/NCCDPHP/publications/AAG/obesity.htm. Accessed May 27, 2009.
2. World Health Organization. Obesity and overweight fact sheet, 2006. Available at: www.who.int/mediacentre/factsheets/fs311/en/index.htm. Accessed May 27, 2009.
3. Ogden CL, Carroll MD, McDowell MA, et al. Obesity among adults in the United States: no change since 2003–2004. NCHS data brief no 1. Hyattsville, MD: National center for health Statistics; 2007.
4. Adams JP, Murphy PG. Obesity in anaesthesia and intensive care. Br J Anaesth 2000;85(1):91–108.
5. Tumuklu MM, Etikan I, Kisacik B, et al. Effect of obesity on left ventricular structure and myocardial systolic function: assessment by tissue Doppler imaging and strain/strain rate imaging. Echocardiography 2007;24(8):802–9.

6. Garret K, Lauer K, Christopher BA. The effects of obesity on the cardiopulmonary system: implications for critical care nursing. Prog Cardiovasc Nurs 2004;19: 155–61.
7. Hu FB. Overweight and obesity in women: health risks and consequences. J Womens Health 2003;12(2):163–72.
8. Maki KC, Kurlandsky S. Syndrome X. A tangled web of risk factors for coronary heart disease and diabetes mellitus. Top Clin Nutr 2001;16(2):32–41.
9. Charlebois D, Wilmoth D. Critical care of patients with obesity. Crit Care Nurse 2004;24(4):19–28.
10. Holm K. Women, heart disease, and obesity. Prog Cardiovasc Nurs 2008;12(2): 163–72, 191–2.
11. Appel SJ, Jones ED, Kennedy-Malone L. Central obesity and the metabolic syndrome: implications for primary care providers. J Am Acad Nurse Pract 2004;16(8):335–42.
12. Coviello JS, Nystrom KV. Obesity and heart failure. J Cardiovasc Nurs 2003;18(5): 360–6.
13. Krishnan R, Becker RJ, Beighley LM, et al. Impact of body mass index on markers of left ventricular thickness and mass calculation: results of a pilot analysis. Echocardiography 2005;22(3):203–10.
14. Haque AK, Gadre S, Taylor J, et al. Pulmonary and cardiovascular complications of obesity. Arch Pathol Lab Med 2008;132:1397–404.
15. Poirier P, Giles TD, Bray GA, et al. Obesity and cardiovascular disease: pathophysiology, evaluation, and effect of weight loss: an update of the 1997 American Heart Association Scientific Statement on Obesity and Heart Disease from the Obesity Committee of the Council on Nutrition, Physical Activity, and Metabolism. Circulation 2006;113:898–918.
16. Joffe A, Wood K. Obesity in critical care. Curr Opin Anaesthesiol 2007;20:113–8.
17. Mihl C, Dassen WRM, Kuipers H. Cardiac remodeling: concentric versus eccentric hypertrophy in strength and endurance athletes. Neth Heart J 2008;16(4): 129–33.
18. Burns SM, Egloff MB, Ryan B, et al. Effect of body position on spontaneous respiratory rate and tidal volume in patients with obesity, abdominal distention and ascites. Am J Crit Care 1994;3:102–6.
19. Harrington L, Leiker C. Dosing of emergency cardiovascular medications in obese patients. Bariatric Nursing and Surgical Patient Care 2007;2(2):131–9.
20. Shibutani K, Inchiosa MAJ, Sawada K, et al. Fentanyl for postoperative analgesia in lean and obese patients. Br J Anaesth 2005;95:377–83.

Pulmonary Aspects of Obesity in Critical Care

Debra Siela, PhD, RN, CCNS, ACNS-BC, CCRN, CNE, RRT [a,b,]*

KEYWORDS

• Obesity • Pulmonary • Critical care • Nursing • Respiratory

More than one third of United States adults were obese in 2005–6 according to the Centers for Disease Control and Prevention (CDC). The prevalence of obesity had increased steadily for 25 years until about 2003. Since that time, the prevalence has not significantly increased. However, the distribution of body mass index (BMI) has shifted to the right over the past 25 years, indicating that the entire adult population is heavier and the heaviest have become heavier.[1]

The CDC reports statistics that demonstrate ever-increasing trends toward a very obese nation.[2] The statistic trends are as follows:

- In 1990, among the states participating in the Behavioral Risk Factor Surveillance System, 10 had a prevalence of obesity less than 10% and no states had prevalence equal to or greater than 15%.
- In 1999, no state had prevalence less than 10%; 18 states had a prevalence of obesity between 20% and 24%; and no state had prevalence equal to or greater than 25%.
- In 2008, only 1 state (Colorado) had a prevalence of obesity less than 20%. Thirty-two states had a prevalence equal to or greater than 25%; 6 of these states (Alabama, Mississippi, Oklahoma, South Carolina, Tennessee, and West Virginia) had a prevalence of obesity equal to or greater than 30%.

The total cost of obesity was $117 billion in the year 2000.[1] In the United States, approximately 300,000 deaths associated with obesity and being overweight occur annually as compared with 400,000 deaths from cigarettes.[1] In addition, the morbidity of obesity affects many types of heart disease, diabetes, cancer, arthritis, reproductive complications, and breathing problems.[3]

BMI is used as an indicator for body fatness. BMI is calculated with a formula that includes dividing weight by height. Normal BMI is 18.5 to 24.9.[4] A BMI of 25 to 30 is rated as overweight, while a BMI greater than 30 is considered to be mild obesity. A BMI between 35 and 35.9 is rated as severe obesity. Morbid obesity is defined as BMI greater than 40.[4]

[a] Ball State University, School of Nursing, 2000 University Avenue, Muncie, IN 47306, USA
[b] Ball Memorial Hospital, Critical Care, 2401 University Avenue, Muncie, IN 47303, USA
* Ball State University, School of Nursing, 2000 University Avenue, Muncie, IN 47306, USA.
E-mail address: dsiela@bsu.edu

Crit Care Nurs Clin N Am 21 (2009) 301–310
doi:10.1016/j.ccell.2009.07.015
0899-5885/09/$ – see front matter © 2009 Elsevier Inc. All rights reserved.

Obese patients are likely to enter and be admitted to critical care nursing units because they are much more susceptible than other patients to thromboembolic disease, myocardial infarction, respiratory failure requiring mechanical ventilation, sepsis, and wound complications.[5] Once they are admitted to a critical care unit, patients who are obese or have a BMI greater than 30 are more likely to experience complications and mortality than those who have a BMI less than 30.[4,6]

One of the biggest challenges of providing care for morbidly obese patients who are critically ill are issues related to the pulmonary system. Morbid obesity affects the pulmonary system in adverse ways. To determine and provide appropriate care for critically ill obese patients, nurses must first understand pulmonary pathophysiology associated with morbid obesity. Pulmonary assessment and pulmonary function is compromised in critically ill patients who are morbidly obese and the compromise increases as the BMI and weight increases.

PATHOPHYSIOLOGY

Lung volumes are reduced in obese persons because the diaphragm is cephaloid-displaced by the obese abdomen, particularly in the supine position.[6,7] These volume reductions are not pronounced in mild obesity, but much more so in morbid obesity.[6]

Small airways and alveoli collapse cause atelectasis, which contributes to poor gas exchange and hypoxemia. Fatty infiltration of respiratory muscles may decrease maximum respiratory pressures, aggravate the abnormal lung volumes, and inhibit the capacity to respond to the increased work of breathing (WOB).[8] Fatigue occurs from the increased use of respiratory muscles and the greatly increased oxygen consumption for these muscles to work.

PULMONARY ASSESSMENT OF OBESE PATIENTS

To make a pulmonary assessment of an obese patient, begin by obtaining a detailed medical history that includes information regarding sleep, snoring, pulmonary disorder, dyspnea, fatigue, cough, and secretions indicative of compromised pulmonary status.[9] The combination of thoracic kyphosis, lumbar lordosis, an elevated diaphragm, and layers of fat on the chest and abdominal walls causes significant decreases in chest movement and lung volumes. The declines in lung volumes are frequently reflected in pulmonary function tests that indicate a restrictive pattern.[9]

Morbid obesity decreases the quality of a portable chest radiograph and obscures the distinction between pneumonic infiltrates and pulmonary edema.[10] Excessive mediastinal adipose tissue projects an abnormal mediastinum on plain chest radiograph, mimicking thoracic aortic aneurysm. Provided the scanner table is strong enough, a CT scan can be performed. A CT scan offers improved visualization of the pulmonary parenchyma and the surrounding vasculature.[10]

Be sure to assess oxygenation, ventilation, and acid-base balance in patients with morbid obesity. Hahler[11] recommends adaptation during pulmonary assessment of morbidly obese patients. Listen for breath sounds by displacing all skin folds over the area and placing the stethoscope diaphragm over the exposed areas. Listen over dependent areas of the lung where fluid may collect and lung tissue is close to the chest wall.

PULMONARY FUNCTION

Reduced lung volumes in obesity include forced vital capacity, functional residual capacity (FRC), total lung capacity, expiratory reserve volume, and maximal voluntary ventilation.[8,12] The most common reduced volumes are FRC and expiratory reserve volume.[8] In patients with a BMI greater than 40, forced vital capacity is reduced by 25% to 50% and maximal voluntary ventilation by 30%.[6] In obesity hypoventilation syndrome (OHS), sometimes known as obstructive sleep apnea, the volumes are even further reduced.[6] Vital capacity and total lung capacity are reduced by 20% to 30% in morbidly obese patients.[8] In addition, FRC is reduced when obese patients are in a supine position.[9]

Reduced FRC eventually results in closing volumes that are larger than closing capacity. The large closing volumes cause closure of small airways even at resting ventilation (tidal ventilation), and these become nonventilated alveoli. Since these non-ventilated alveoli are still perfused, there is ventilation-to-perfusion mismatch and right-to-left shunt.[9] Maximal voluntary ventilation is low in obesity because of high WOB and high energy-cost of breathing.[7] In addition, respiratory rate is higher in obese patients by 40%.[6]

COMPLIANCE

Respiratory system compliance decreases exponentially as a function of increased BMI.[8] Both lung tissue and chest wall compliance are reduced in obesity because of the excess adipose tissue.[6] Compliance is decreased by 25% in simple obesity and by 40% in OHS. Regional changes in chest wall compliance may be a factor in prone versus supine improvement in oxygenation.[6]

AIRWAY RESISTANCE

Reduced lung volume due to unventilated alveoli and closed small airways contributes to increased airway resistance.[6] Increased airway resistance in small airways in patients with severe to morbid obesity is likely due to increased abdominal pressure and small lung volume.[9]

GAS EXCHANGE

Morbidly obese patients are prone to hypoxemia because of low lung volumes.[13] In addition, because the diaphragm protrudes upward into the chest and decreases the size of thorax, Po_2 is likely low in supine positions. The main cause of hypoxemia is ventilation-perfusion mismatch due to poor ventilation of the alveoli in the lung bases. Perfusion of the alveoli in the bases is usually adequate.

Pelosi and colleagues[6] examined body mass effects on lung volumes, respiratory mechanics, and gas exchange in patients during general anesthesia. They found that when BMI increased, oxygenation index (ratio of partial pressure of oxygen, arterial [Pao_2] to partial pressure of oxygen in the alveoli [Pao_2]) decreased and correlated with the FRC.

Carbon dioxide production increases as a function of body weight. However, in normal patients, the increase per kilogram is 40% higher than it is in obese patients.[7] The respiratory quotient or Vco_2/Vo_2 is normal for most obese patients. Most obese patients remain eucapnic unless they also have OHS, in which case they also become hypercapnic.[7]

WORK OF BREATHING AND OXYGEN COST OF BREATHING

The WOB is performed by the respiratory muscles to expand the chest wall and the lung.[14] The respiratory muscles must overcome elastic and nonelastic forces of compliance and resistance. When compliance decreases or resistance increases, more force is required to move a volume of gas in the lung, thus increasing the WOB.[13] Patients with simple obesity breathe about 40% faster than patients of normal weight.[8] WOB is increased because of the increased abdominal fat mass and increased elastic and resistive loads.[8] The WOB is 60% higher in simple obesity and as much as 250% higher in morbid obesity.[8]

The oxygen cost of breathing increases for simple obesity to as much as five times normal and for OHS to about 10 times normal.[8] Oxygen consumption increases linearly with weight, and most obese patients have a resting hypoxemia. Because the excess fat increases metabolic activity, carbon dioxide production and the need for its elimination are also increased. The combination of these effects requires that obese patients have a higher minute ventilation to maintain normocarbia. Any further metabolic stress that adds to these oxygen demands, or any further decline in pulmonary function, can quickly lead to respiratory decompensation.[9]

Kress and colleagues[15] determined that morbidly obese patients had significantly higher baseline oxygen consumption (Vo_2) during spontaneous breathing compared with nonobese patients. In addition, these same morbidly obese patients, before receiving mechanical ventilation, also had a significant decrease in Vo_2 when switching from spontaneous breathing to mechanical ventilation. The researchers concluded that morbidly obese patients use a high percentage of their total oxygen consumption just to breathe even at rest because of low respiratory reserve.

DYSPNEA

Dyspnea or breathlessness is uncommon in patients with simple obesity.[8] Patients with severe obesity tend to have reduced diaphragmatic function because of diaphragm overstretching, particularly when in a recumbent position.[8] These severely obese patients usually experience dyspnea. In OHS, inspiratory muscle strength is often reduced and dyspnea is common. Increased WOB contributes to the perception of increased dyspnea or breathlessness.

Sahebjami,[16] after examining healthy obese men with and without dyspnea, found that dyspneic obese men, compared with nondyspneic healthy obese men, had a higher body weight and BMI along with a lower maximal voluntary ventilation and maximum expiratory pressure. These findings are consistent with the perception of dyspnea that often accompanies low lung volumes and low lung reserve with increasing BMI in morbidly obese patients.

Davidson and colleagues[17] suggest the use of a fan over the head of the bed to decrease the sensation of dyspnea. The use of the reverse Trendelenburg position should also aid in decreasing the sensation of dyspnea by allowing space in the thorax for closed compressed alveoli to be ventilated.

AIRWAY MANAGEMENT
Endotracheal Intubation

Intubation of obese patients is often problematic.[18,19] Brodsky and colleagues[20] demonstrated that a large neck circumference and a Mallampati score or classification of 3 (soft and hard palate and base of the uvula are visible) correlated with problematic intubation. Neck circumference greater than 40 cm was associated with a 5% probability of difficult intubation, while a neck circumference of 60 cm was associated with a 35% probability of difficult intubation. The normal neck circumference in a 70-kg man is 35 cm. A neck circumference of 60 cm or greater is associated with a 35% chance of difficult intubation.[20] The larger the neck circumference, the more difficult is the laryngoscopy and intubation.

Mcauliffe and Edge[9] recommend assessing before intubation, if possible, the ability of the obese patient to adequately open his or her mouth and fully extend the neck. Excess cervical fat makes positioning the head in a neutral position difficult. In obese patients, cervical adipose tissue, a large tongue, and a constricted glottic opening all contribute to a narrow upper airway. Also, fat distribution patterns within the soft tissues of the oral airway increase the likelihood that relaxation of airway muscles may lead to collapse of the oropharynx between the uvula and epiglottis. This can cause difficulty in ventilating with a mask. An endotracheal tube may be needed but securing the airway may be more difficult.

El-Solh[10] recommends awake-patient intubation before anesthesia induction. A study by Dixon and colleagues[19] demonstrated that 100% oxygen administered while the head of bed is at a 25° angle before anesthesia improved oxygenation by 23%.

Increased fat disposition and muscle relaxation may cause the oropharynx between the epiglottis and uvula to collapse. In such cases, Brodsky and colleagues[20] recommend intubation with an endotracheal tube in the pharynx. Position patients with the head, upper body, and shoulders significantly elevated above the chest, so that an imaginary horizontal line could connect the patient's sternal notch with his or her external auditory meatus. This ramped positioning resulted in 99 out of 100 successful intubations in morbidly obese patients. Researchers believe that this ramped positioning improves the laryngeal view in obese patients over a 7-cm cushion under the patient's head.[20,21]

Pelosi and colleagues[6] suggest that, to successfully intubate morbidly obese patients, the patients be awake and in a reverse Trendelenburg position. They enumerate five reasons for choosing this method:

1. Patients maintain patency of the natural airways and spontaneous breathing.
2. FRC is not reduced by anesthetics and muscle relaxants; thus oxygenation is preserved.
3. Muscle tone maintains upper airway structures in the usual position so that they are easier to identify.
4. Mask ventilation is not necessary.
5. The reverse Trendelenburg position allows maintenance of approximate physiologic values of FRC, closing volumes, and gas exchange during the procedure. Moreover, this position improves the visual setting during intubation compared with the supine position.

If traditional intubation techniques are unsuccessful, use of fiber-optic intubation may be considered as an alternative means of intubation.

Tracheostomy

Tracheostomy is commonly performed to replace endotracheal tubes as an airway for long-term ventilator-dependent patients. Advantages of tracheostomy over endotracheal tubes include lower airway resistance, smaller dead space, less movement of the tube within the trachea, greater patient comfort, and more efficient secretion control.[21] However, tracheostomies are also associated with serious complications, such as tracheal stenosis, increased bacterial colonization, and fatal hemorrhage.[22]

El Solh and Jaafar[23] conducted a comparative study of tracheostomy complications. They reported that morbidly obese patients with tracheostomies experienced significantly more complications than nonmorbidly obese patients in the control group. The complication rate for morbidly obese patients was 25% versus 14% for nonmorbidly obese patients in the control group. The most serious or life-threatening complications were related to loss of airway accessibility. Thus, conducting frequent assessment, monitoring, and care of the tracheostomy airway is necessary to prevent, identify, and treat serious tracheostomy complications of the morbidly obese patient.

If a tracheostomy is buried deep in fatty tissue, a large wound increases risk of bleeding, infection, or damage of the surrounding tissue, need to protect the peristomal skin, manage the tracheostomy, and contain wound drainage.[23–25] Patients may need specially sized tracheostomy tubes that have enough length to traverse the diameter of the neck wall.[11] In addition, narrow cloth ties can burrow into the neck folds, impairing skin and tissue integrity of the neck. Tracheostomy ties likely need to be thicker and wider than normal.[11]

A percutaneous dilational tracheostomy (PDT) is a type of tracheostomy procedure that can be performed at the bedside.[16] A small incision is made in the neck and trachea. The opening is enlarged using specialized dilators until the desired tracheostomy tube can fit into the opening. This procedure requires no anesthesia, does not need to be performed in an operating room, and results in fewer complications than comparable procedures. Patients who might not be candidates for PDT include those requiring high levels of ventilator support, those with neck problems, and those who are obese.

However, PDT may be a viable option as an airway for morbidly obese patients. Masharamani and colleagues[26] performed PDT on 13 morbidly obese patients. These clinical investigators determined that PDT was a safe and successful procedure for morbidly obese patients requiring a tracheostomy.

VENTILATION ASSISTANCE

Morbid obesity has been associated with prolonged mechanical ventilation, extended weaning periods, and longer lengths of stay in intensive care units and hospitals.[10] Reasons for delayed liberation from mechanical ventilation were attributed to the increased WOB and suboptimal lung mechanics.

The role of increased intra-abdominal pressure in reducing FRC in obese patients has been described. Increased intra-abdominal pressure results in decreased respiratory compliance and oxygenation with relevant collapse and atelectasis. To ventilate obese patients during anesthesia in the operating room, one must compensate for increased intra-abdominal pressure that reduces FRC. Four different modalities of ventilation have been proposed. These include high inspiratory oxygen fractions; ventilation using tidal volume as high as 15 to 20 mL/kg ideal body weight; inclusion of large, manually or automatically performed lung inflations (sighs); and application of positive end-expiratory pressure (PEEP) after a recruitment maneuver. The investigators state that these modalities have not been compared with each other in a research investigation.

Based upon their research and experience, Pelosi and colleagues[6] stated that, to ventilate lungs that tend to collapse in obese patients, inspiratory pressures must be high enough to recruit the collapsed alveoli. This would require using a PEEP high enough to keep the lung open at end expiration associated with low tidal volumes and fraction of inspired oxygen (Fio_2) lower than 0.8. They proposed the following mechanical ventilation management guidelines during surgery:

- Tidal volume 6 to 10 mL/kg ideal body weight and respiratory rate to maintain normocapnia
- Recruitment maneuver (40–60 cm) over 6 seconds, three times in pressure or volume control) once hemodynamic stability has been obtained and volemia is stable after induction of anesthesia
- Application of PEEP 10 cm H_2O always after a recruitment maneuver

- Reverse Trendelenburg position (35°) when possible
- F_{IO_2} between 0.4 and 0.8

In the postoperative period, consider application of continuous positive airway pressure by helmet or mask if mechanical ventilation is not required and when P_{O_2}/F_{IO_2} falls below 300.[6] PEEP should be used in obesity to recruit alveoli and reduce atelectasis.[7] If mechanical ventilation is required, tidal volume should be calculated according to the patient's ideal body weight and not his or her actual weight.[27]

POSITIONING

The optimal position of a morbidly obese patient is one that prevents excessive abdominal pressure against the diaphragm and allows adequate diaphragmatic excursion. Burns and colleagues[27] conducted a study in which critically ill patients with large abdomens on mechanical ventilator support were placed in several different positions related to head-of-bed elevation. The best position that resulted in the largest tidal volume and lowest respiratory rate was the 45° reverse Trendelenburg. This position appeared to facilitate the weaning process by optimizing lung mechanics. Reverse Trendelenburg position allows the abdomen to drop down and away from the thoracic cavity, promoting diaphragmatic excursion.

The gastric volume of the stomach is larger in patients who are obese than in patients who are not obese.[28] The large panniculus and increased intra-abdominal fat in patients who are obese result in high intra-abdominal pressures, thus increasing the risk of gastric reflux and pulmonary aspiration. Head-of-bed elevation may decrease intra-abdominal pressures and allow the diaphragm to be in its normal position. Patients with obesity should be placed in the reverse Trendelenburg position at 45° after their hemodynamic status is stabilized.

NURSING AND RESPIRATORY CARE

Goals of nursing and respiratory care are to promote an effective breathing pattern and gas exchange for critically ill obese patients. Garrett and colleagues[29] recommend that nurses should:

Avoid supine, lithotomy, and Trendelenburg positions
Assess for clinical signs of hypoxia, including altered level of consciousness, dysrhythmias, cyanosis, and changes in rate, depth, or quality of respirations
Monitor pulse oximetry and arterial blood gases

In addition, use of specialty beds with lateral rotation should also be considered to assist in mobilizing secretions and improving ventilation.[24] Nurses must also provide appropriate airway management, including oral care. See tracheostomy section.

Repositioning and moving the morbidly obese patient is important to promote full lung ventilation and prevent complications of immobility.[25] Davidson and colleagues[17] advises that a regular schedule of manual turning and repositioning is necessary. Turning obese patients requires many staff members. Up to five people may be required to safely lift and reposition an unconscious morbidly obese patient. Davidson and colleagues[17] suggest adding hours per care to the acuity system for the care of a morbidly obese patient. They estimate that care of the unconscious or full-care morbidly obese patient may require an additional 1.5 hours of care.

Morbidly obese patients who are awake and can participate in their care should be mobilized to prevent pulmonary and other systemic complications. Davidson and colleagues[17] recommend the use of beds that can be raised to a sitting position and then, by removing the footboard, allow the patient to walk out the end of the bed.

Because morbidly obese patients have multiple skin folds, they must be inspected during every turn session. This includes the folds behind the neck where endotracheal or tracheostomy tube tape or ties reside. The posterior neck area of a morbidly obese patient with folds and endotracheal tube tape is at high risk for impaired skin integrity.[11] In addition, saliva and sputum commonly collects in the posterior neck area, contributing to the risk of impaired skin integrity.

PHARMACOLOGY ISSUES OF CRITICALLY ILL OBESE PATIENTS

Patients who are obese have a high fat-to-muscle ratio. Muscle tissue holds more water than does fat tissue.[28] As a result, drugs with hydrophilic distribution properties may be distributed into part, but not all, of the adipose tissue.

Critically ill obese patients must be assessed frequently for anxiolytic, analgesic, and antidepressant needs. Many drugs in these classifications are lipophilic and are taken up by adipose tissue and released slowly into the blood.

The intravenous and enteral routes are preferred for administration of medications in patients with obesity. Adipose tissue has a decreased blood supply, and drugs given by the subcutaneous route have a delayed onset of action and an unpredictable duration of action. Similarly, transdermal patches are a poor choice for delivery of medications in patients who are obese. Onset of action of transdermal-delivered medications is delayed in patients who are obese, and duration of drug action is erratic and unpredictable.

SUMMARY

Critically ill obese patients have many challenging pulmonary problems. The first key is to understand pathophysiology in the pulmonary system related to obesity. Second, it is important to identify the altered physical assessments and diagnostics that occur because of the pulmonary pathophysiology of obesity. Lastly, one should be aware of medical and nursing intervention options that treat symptoms or pulmonary problems of obesity.

REFERENCES

1. U.S. Department of Health and Human Services. Overweight and obesity threaten U.S. health gains. Communities can help address the problem, surgeon general says. Available at: http://www.cdc.gov/nchs/data/databriefs/db01.pdf. Accessed February 28, 2009.
2. Centers for Disease Control and Prevention. U.S. obesity trends 1985–2008. Available at: http://www.cdc.gov/obesity/data/trends.html. Accessed February 28, 2009.
3. U.S. Department of Health & Human Services-Office of the Surgeon General. Overweight and obesity: health consequences. Available at: http://www.surgeongeneral.gov/topics/obesity/calltoaction/fact_consequences.html. Accessed February 28, 2009.
4. Centers for Disease Control and Prevention. About BMI for adults. Available at: http://www.cdc.gov/healthyweight/assessing/bmi/adult_bmi/index.html. Accessed February 28, 2009.

5. Bercault N, Boulain T, Kuteifan K, et al. Obesity-related excess mortality rate in an adult intensive care unit: a risk-adjusted matched cohort study. Crit Care Med 2004;324:998–1003.
6. Pelosi P, Luecke T, Caironi P, et al. A physiologic based approach to perioperative management of obese patients. In: Albert R, Slutsky A, Ranier M, et al, editors. Clinical critical care medicine. Philadelphia: Mosby Elsevier; 2006.
7. Guerin C, Koutsoukou A, Milic-Emili J, et al. Lung mechanics in disease. In: Papadakos P, Lachmann B, editors. Mechanical ventilation: clinical applications and pathophysiology. Philadelphia: Saunders Elsevier; 2008.
8. Tzelepis G, McCool D. The lungs and chest wall disease. In: Mason R, Broaddus V, Murray J, editors. Murray and Nadel's textbook of respiratory medicine. 4th edition. Philadelphia: Saunders Elsevier; 2005.
9. Mcauliffe M, Edge M. Perioperative and anesthesia considerations in obese patients. Bariatric Nursing and Surgical Patient Care 2007;2:123–30.
10. El-Soh A. Clinical approach to the critically ill, morbidly obese patient. Am J Respir Crit Care Med 2004;169:557–61.
11. Hahler B. Morbid obesity: a nursing care challenge. MedSurg Nursing 2002; 11(2):85–90.
12. Jones R, Nzekwn M. The effects of body mass index on lung volumes. Chest 2003;130(3):827–33.
13. Biring M, Lewis M, Liu J, et al. Pulmonary physiologic changes of morbid obesity. Am J Med Sci 1999;318:293–7.
14. Pierce L. Management of the mechanically ventilated patient. 2nd edition. St. Louis (MO): Saunders Elsevier; 2007.
15. Kress J, Pohlman A, Alverdy J, et al. The impact of morbid obesity on oxygen cost of breathing (VO_{2RESP}) at rest. Am J Respir Crit Care Med 1999;160:883–6.
16. Sahebjami H. Dyspnea in obese healthy men. Chest 1998;114:1373–7.
17. Davidson J, Kruse M, Cox D, et al. Critical care of the morbidly obese. Critical Care Nurse Quarterly 2003;26(2):105–6.
18. Waltz J, Zayaruzny M, Heard S. Airway management in critical illness. Chest 2007;131:608–20.
19. Dixon B, Dixon J, Carden J, et al. Preoxygenation is more effective in the 25 degrees head-up position than in the supine position in severely obese patients: a randomized controlled study. Anesthesiology 2005;102:1110–5.
20. Brodsky J, Lemmons H, Brock-Utne J, et al. Morbid obesity and tracheal intubation. Anesth Analg 2002;94:732–6.
21. Brodsky J, Lemmens H, Brock-Utne J, et al. Anesthetic considerations for bariatric surgery: proper positioning is important for laryngoscopy. Anesth Analg 2003; 96:1841–2.
22. Collins J, Lemmons H, Brodsky J, et al. Laryngoscopy and morbid obesity: a comparision of the "sniff" and "ramped" positions. Obes Surg 2004;14:1171–5.
23. El Solh A, Jaafar W. A comparative study of the complications of surgical tracheostomy in morbidly obese critically ill paitents. Crit Care 2007;11(1):1–6.
24. Gallagher S. Obesity and the skin in the critical care setting. Crit Care Nurs 2002; 25(1):69–75.
25. Marik P, Varon J. The obese patient in the ICU. Chest 1998;113:492–8.
26. Mansharamani NG, Koziel H, Garland R, et al. Safety of bedside percutaneous dilatational tracheostomy in obese patients in the ICU. Chest 2000;117:1426–9.
27. Burns SM, Egloff MB, Ryan B, et al. Effect of body position on spontaneous respiratory rate and tidal volume in patients with obesity, abdominal distention, and ascites. Am J Crit Care 1994;3:102–6.

28. Charlebois D, Wilmoth D. Critical care of patients with obesity. Crit Care Nurse 2004;24(4):19–29.
29. Garrett K, Lauer K, Christopher BA. The effects of obesity on the cardiopulmonary system: implications for critical care nursing. Prog Cardiovasc Nurs 2004;19: 155–61.

Skin Integrity in Critically Ill Obese Patients

Jeanne Redlin Lowe, PhD(C), RN, CWCN *

KEYWORDS

- Obesity • Bariatric • Skin • Wound • Critical care
- Pressure ulcer

More than 400 million adults worldwide were classified by the World Health Organization (WHO) as obese in 2005, with a projected increase to 700 million by 2015.[1] Obesity is the fastest growing chronic condition in the United States, affecting greater than 30% of the adult population.[2] For the age group of 40–59 year olds, the obesity prevalence is over 40%.[3] Minority women are disproportionately affected, with greater than 50% of non-Hispanic black women and Mexican-American women ages 40–59 being obese.[4] In critical care, these statistics are replicated, with almost one-third of intensive care unit (ICU) patients being obese.[5,6] Obese patients are more likely to have increased lengths of stay, higher morbidity, and increased likelihood of discharge to nursing home facilities.[6–9] Obese patients also pose a unique challenge for preventing skin breakdown, healing wounds, and preventing complications of surgery and prolonged immobility. Yet little research to date has been done to study the effects of obesity on skin integrity and wound healing in this patient population.

Many challenges are presented with care of the obese patient in the intensive care unit. Difficulties with mobilization and re-positioning, unpredictability of pharmacokinetic effects,[7] and lack of appropriate diagnostic equipment to monitor hypotension, hypoxia, and hypoperfusion put these patients at increased risk for skin breakdown and wound healing problems. There are many associated diseases that go along with being overweight and obese.[3]

These co-morbidities – especially diabetes, hypertension, cardiovascular disease, and pulmonary dysfunction – not only make obese patients sicker when they come to the ICU, they also may make them more prone to skin breakdown and wound healing complications while they are there.[6]

Critical care patients who are overweight or obese are at much higher risk of systemic inflammatory response syndrome (SIRS) leading to multiple organ

School of Nursing, Biobehavioral Nursing and Health Systems, Box 357266, University of Washington, Seattle, WA 98195, USA

* Corresponding author.

E-mail address: jlowe@u.washington.edu

Crit Care Nurs Clin N Am 21 (2009) 311–322
doi:10.1016/j.ccell.2009.07.007
0899-5885/09/$ – see front matter © 2009 Elsevier Inc. All rights reserved.

dysfunction syndrome (MODS).[5,10,11] Hypotension, hypoxia, and hypoperfusion are endpoints of MODS that decrease tissue perfusion and increase a patient's risk of skin breakdown. Newell and colleagues (2007) stratified risk of pressure ulcer development in critically ill patients by body mass index (BMI) and found that risk for pressure ulcer compared with patients of normal BMI was more than 1.5 times greater for patients with BMI 30 to 39.9, and almost threefold greater for patients with BMI greater than or equal to 40. Factors that influence skin breakdown, such as sedation, use of paralytics, fluid overload, fever, incontinence, and mechanical trauma are especially important to assess in the obese critical care patient.

Obese patients often have a history of previous discrimination or embarrassment when seeking health care. As a result they may delay seeking care until they are very sick. Impaired body image also makes them less likely to perform recommended self-examinations. A recent study found that obese women with poor body satisfaction were less likely to perform skin examinations for melanoma detection.[8] Therefore, presenting disease states may be more advanced than patients of normal weight.

During skin assessments and wound care, it is especially important that staff be aware of the potential for the patient to feel exposed. Care should be taken not to make the patient feel as if they are a spectacle or on display. Staff attitude about caring for obese patients can be easily transmitted to the patient, and it can be detrimental to a patient's care if the patient feels like the staff resents caring for them or is repulsed by their body habitus.

COMMON SKIN CONDITIONS AND CHRONIC WOUNDS ASSOCIATED WITH OBESITY

There are many skin conditions and chronic wounds associated with obesity.[9,12] Patients who are critically ill may present to the ICU as a result of complications of these skin conditions, or they may be coincidentally treated for them while hospitalized for another medical problem.

Diabetic Foot Ulcers

Almost 24 million adults in the United States have diabetes, and obesity is one of the main risk factors for Type II diabetes.[10] Diabetic foot ulcers occur in about 15% of patients with diabetes.[11] Foot ulcers and infections are one of the top reasons for diabetic patient admission to the hospital.[13] Osteomyelitis, amputation, or death can occur from a diabetic foot ulcer.[14–16] Aggressive treatment of a diabetic foot ulcer including surgical debridement and systemic antibiotics is required in a patient with signs of decreased perfusion and/or sepsis.[17]

Venous Insufficiency Ulcers

Chronic venous insufficiency or venous hypertension of the lower limbs is common in obese people. Danielsson, and colleagues (2002)[18] showed that there was a significant association between BMI and increased clinical severity of chronic venous disease. Patients who were overweight were much more likely to have skin changes and ulceration. The authors concluded that being overweight appears to be a separate risk factor for increased severity of alterations in skin integrity in patients with chronic venous disease. The "gold standard" for treatment of lower limb venous insufficiency is compression via either garments or dressings.[19,20] In the critical care unit, ace wraps are easy to apply and remove and can be used to decrease edema by promoting venous return. Elevation of the lower extremities also aids venous return.

Lymphedema

Lymphedema is caused by dilation of lymph tissue channels when lymph drainage is impaired. Lymphatic fluid accumulates and causes swelling, decreased tissue perfusion and leakage of protein-rich lymphatic fluid into surrounding tissue Bacterial infections are common and permanent tissue changes are manifested by hyperkeratosis (skin thickening). Treatment for lymphedema while the patient is in the critical care unit should be directed at reducing limb size, promoting lymph drainage, and preventing infection. Cellulitis and skin breakdown in the critical care patient with lymphedema can be avoided by daily cleansing with mild soap and water, using compression stockings or ace wraps, and elevating the affected limb.

Intertrigo

Intertrigo is caused by friction between skin surfaces, and usually presents as mild erythema. Frequent sites of intertrigo are skin folds and areas that retain heat and moisture such as: posterior neck, axilla, under breasts, under pannus, perineal area, and inner thighs.[9,21] More severe intertrigo shows signs of inflammation, maceration, and erosion. Secondary bacterial and fungal infections such as candidiasis are common and should be treated by keeping skin folds dry and with topical antimicrobials. Barrier ointments that contain zinc oxide can aid the drying process. Bulky dressings or linen should not be placed in skin folds, since they may contribute to pressure necrosis of the skin.

Psoriasis

Psoriasis is a chronic inflammatory skin condition that has been associated with the secretion of proinflammatory cytokines.[22] Rapid cell turnover causes plaques to form anywhere on the body. Multiple studies have shown an increased correlation between obesity, metabolic syndrome, cardiovascular risk and psoriasis.[23–26] Setty, and colleagues (2007)[23] used prospective data from the Nurses' Health Study II to show the increased incidence of psoriasis in women with higher BMI. Relative risk for psoriasis in nurses with a BMI $\geq$ 30 was 1.73 (95% CI, 1.24–2.41) compared with 0.76 (95% CI, 0.65–0.90) for nurses with a BMI < 21. There are many topical and systemic treatments for psoriasis. Psoriasis is a lifelong disorder, so patients will typically have a history of what has worked for them when they have a flare up.

Perineal Dermatitis

Incontinence of bowel and bladder in obese patients is a common cause of perineal dermatitis which can increase tissue friability and place patients at higher risk for skin breakdown.[27,28] Gentle cleansing after each incontinent episode and the use of barrier creams to protect skin is recommended.[21,29,30]

Pressure Ulcers

According to research by the National Pressure Ulcer Advisory Panel (NPUAP), up to 40% of patients will develop a pressure ulcer while in critical care units.[27] Risk assessment scales for skin breakdown such as the Braden Risk Assessment Scale have been validated in many different patient populations, yet none specifically have been tested in obese patients.[28] The Braden Scale assesses risk for pressure ulcer development based on six patient characteristics: sensory perception, moisture, activity, mobility, nutrition, and friction/shear – with total score ranging from 6 to 23. A score of 16 or less indicates risk for pressure ulcer development. Interventions to prevent skin breakdown should address specific characteristics that put the patient at risk. Risk assessment should be performed on admission to the ICU and at least every 48 hours, or according to changes in the patient's condition.[31,32]

According to the NPUAP definition, "a pressure ulcer is localized injury to the skin and/or underlying tissue usually over a bony prominence, as a result of pressure, or pressure in combination with shear and/or friction."[33] Pressure ulcers in obese patients can also occur in uncommon areas. The weight of adipose tissue can cause enough pressure to occlude capillaries and lead to decreased tissue perfusion and injury. Careful attention should be given to patient skin folds areas such as under breasts (for both genders), beneath the pannus, in perineal and gluteal folds, lumbar and mid-back areas, and posterior neck. Small equipment and tubing used on patients should be carefully monitored to prevent skin breakdown. Pressure ulcer development from foley catheter tubing, tracheostomy ties, endotracheal tube holders or other equipment left under patients can occur.

Pressure ulcers are staged according to depth of injury.[29] The increased tissue load of obesity can lead to more serious tissue injury.[24,25] Kraemer-Aguiar and colleagues[30] (2008) studied skin microcirculatory dysfunction in diabetic patients with increased body mass index. They found that patients with increased BMI had smaller afferent, efferent, and apical capillary diameters; lower functional capillary density; less capillaries per square millimeter; and less red blood cell velocity; all leading to longer time to reach post-occlusive reactive hyperemia. Tissue perfusion is decreased for longer periods of time in obese patients when their tissue is subjected to pressure. As a result, obese patients may be more susceptible to pressure-related tissue injuries related to their size.

Elsner and Gefen (2008) studied the development of deep tissue injury (DTI) in patients with spinal cord injury (SCI) who are obese. Their study observed average increases of 1.5 times of stresses on internal soft tissues (muscle, fat) over bony prominences with a rise in BMI from 25.5 to 40 kg/m^2.[34] The authors also noted that muscle atrophy associated with SCI combined with the increased bodyweight led to increased tissue loads that increased the likelihood of deep tissue injury.

Several studies in critical care have shown that guideline concurrent care for prevention and treatment of pressure ulcers can impact their prevalence and incidence.[35–38] However, implementation of pressure ulcer prevention and treatment guidelines in the critically ill obese population is often difficult.

Ability to turn - given the patient's clinical condition, appropriate equipment, and adequate staffing levels - can affect the ability to assess, prevent, and treat pressure ulcers. Tissue injury in skin folds or on posterior surfaces of the body may be difficult to assess in larger patients. Consequently, progression of tissue injury to necrosis may occur more frequently in obese patients. In critical care, there are also conflicting priorities of positioning the patient for optimal ventilation versus. preventing shearing injuries. By keeping the head of the bed greater than 30 degrees, as is required by most guidelines to prevent ventilator acquired pneumonia (VAP),[39] intubated patients are at higher risk for sliding down in bed, thus subjecting them to shearing forces on their posterior skin.[19] Gatching the knees of the bed frame before elevating the head of the bed may prevent some sliding and reduce potential for shearing injuries.

Guideline concurrent care also indicates that patients at risk for developing pressure ulcers should be placed on pressure reduction surfaces.[21,29,30] However, access to size-appropriate pressure reduction surfaces may be limited. In addition, staff knowledge about suitable mattress selections for the obese patient is often lacking. Several companies now offer for sale or rent pressure reduction mattresses and overlays that can accommodate patients up to 1,000 pounds. It is often more cost-effective for hospitals to purchase these surfaces, given the growing population of critically ill obese patients.

Poor nutrition is another risk factor for skin breakdown and pressure ulcer development.[31–33] Obese patients are frequently malnourished since their weight may be due to increased ingestion of high-density energy foods that are high in fat and sugars but low in vitamins, minerals and other micronutrients.[1,29] To promote wound healing and prevent complications from protein depletion, it is imperative to prevent catabolic states. To estimate calorie requirements, energy expenditure must be assessed. Anthropometric assessment of caloric requirements using indirect calorimetry is one way to assess calorie requirements, but it is expensive, and the equipment is not readily available in some hospital settings. Estimation of metabolic rates can also be done using caloric calculations. The Penn State equation for estimating energy expenditure has been validated in critically ill obese patients under age 60.[20] It is calculated using the patient's basal metabolic rate, minute ventilation, and maximum temperature. Based on these calculations, patients should be fed early or have parenteral or enteral feeding started to prevent catabolic states.

Wound healing involves anabolic metabolism and will not occur without adequate protein stores. Infections, wounds, and stress all increase metabolic requirements.[40] Immune mediators are protein based and quickly depleted by protein malnourishment and healing demands. Protein stores can be evaluated by assessing the patient's serum albumin, pre-albumin, and/or transthyretin levels.[19,20] Nitrogen balance to assess for catabolic metabolism can also be evaluated by a 24 hour urine collection.

SURGICAL WOUND COMPLICATIONS IN OBESE PATIENTS

Post-surgical wound complications are also very common in obese patients. In a retrospective study of a cohort of patients receiving post-bariatric surgery, Arthurs, and colleagues (2007)[41] found that patients with a BMI > 25 kg/m^2 were three times as likely to have post-operative wound complications. Another study of patients undergoing bariatric surgery found that very obese patients were at risk for post-operative necrosis of their gluteal muscles, with subsequent renal failure and death, related to their BMI.[42]

Infections

There is inadequate information about dosing antibiotics in the obese patient and limited data on pharmokinetic differences.[43,44] Data that we do have are from small case-based studies.[12,45] As a result, obese patients may be more prone to surgical infections due to sub-therapeutic antibiotic levels. Pinsolle and colleagues (2006)[14] analyzed records over a 12-year period of women receiving breast reconstruction. They found that surgical infections were more likely to occur in obese women, and for that reason they recommended that reconstruction be delayed or contraindicated in patients that were obese.

Fournier's gangrene is a necrotizing soft tissue infection of the perineum that can occur in either gender. Predisposing risk factors for these infections include diabetes, obesity, and immunocompromise.[15] Patients often are admitted to the hospital ICU with advanced infections, sepsis, and shock. Treatment includes systemic antibiotics and supportive therapy, serial surgical debridement, and daily wound care.

Graft Failure

Skin grafting is usually required for definitive wound closure of large tissue defects caused by conditions such as Fournier's gangrene and other post-surgical wounds.

However, graft failure in the obese patient is common,[16] and patients are often left with huge chronic wounds healing via secondary intention.

Incision Dehiscence and Seroma Formation

Other common post-surgical sequelae in obese patients that complicate wound healing include incision dehiscence[46,47] and seroma or hematoma formation.[48] Incisional dehiscence is often due to mechanical failure caused by increased tension on tissue at the incision site, infections, and inadequate nutrition. Use of supportive garments such as abdominal binders, systemic treatment of infection, and nutritional interventions may improve incisional wound healing and decrease incidence of dehiscence.

Seroma formation in patients post skin excision is associated with the amount of tissue removed.[48] Seroma and hematoma development under surgical sites can also lead to incision wound failures, but can be effectively treated with aspiration of fluid and/or proper placement of wound drains.[49]

WOUND MANAGEMENT

While guidelines for general wound management are not specifically targeted to obese patients in the ICU, the evidence-based principles for prevention and wound healing should be followed when caring for critically ill obese patients with wounds.[31,50–53]

Pain Control

Pain control during wound care is important, but dosing of pain medication in obese patients can be unpredictable due to variations in absorption rates.[31] Increased adipose tissue in obese patients makes the use of lipophilic drugs for pain control problematic. Lipophilic analgesics may be sequestered in adipose tissue and cause re-sedation syndrome with subsequent respiratory depression.[54] Hydrophilic drugs that are water soluble and distributed in lean tissue (calculated using ideal body weight) should be the drugs of choice for pain control during wound care to prevent post-procedural sedation and respiratory depression.[43] Less lipophilic analgesics such as fentanyl or morphine should be used. Titration of dose to effect should be monitored closely.[44] Administration of analgesia should be via oral or intravenous routes, since drugs given via transdermal, subcutaneous, and intramuscular routes all have unpredictable absorption in patients with excess adipose tissue.

Dressing Selection

Wound management protocols for obese patients often involve pre-planning and multidisciplinary coordination of care.[52–54] Access to the affected area of the body often present challenges for wound assessment and dressing changes. Appropriate staffing and equipment can facilitate wound care and decrease injury to staff and patients. Limb slings for use with lift equipment are available for caring for wounds of the lower extremities. Wound dressings in appropriate size selections for larger patients should be readily accessible.

Palliative Wound Care

According to guidelines on palliative care in the intensive care unit from the American College of Critical Care Medicine (2008) iatrogenic sources of pain such as wound care should be minimized or eliminated.[45] Patients who are at end-of-life often have wounds. Focus should shift from healing the wounds to providing comfort and symptom management by controlling pain and managing infection, odor, bleeding, and drainage.[55,56]

OTHER CONSIDERATIONS
Mobilizing Obese Patients in the ICU

A recent nationwide survey of physical therapists who work in critical care areas noted that only 10% of critical care units have established criteria for the initiation of physical therapy, and that 89% of the hospitals required a physician order to initiate therapy.[57] Mobilizing obese critical care patients can be especially difficult due to their size. Specialized equipment and additional staffing is often required for patients over 250 pounds. Yet complications of immobility such as lost muscle mass, atelectasis and pneumonia, and skin breakdown are especially critical to course of the hospital stay for the obese ICU patient.

Utilizing appropriate equipment and interdisciplinary protocols when caring for obese patients can improve mobility and decrease skin breakdown.[58,59] Representatives from departments across the continuum of care should provide input on protocol development.[58] A patient or family representative should also contribute their perspective to promote patient-centered care.

Equipment Needs

Traditionally, most hospital equipment was not built to hold patients greater than 250 pounds. Wall-mounted toilets have broken off walls when used by patients over that weight limit – sometimes injuring the patient in the process. Emergency room staff has resorted to tying gurneys together to accommodate obese patients. Obese patients have been crammed into regular sized hospital beds that make re-positioning impossible. It is important to know the weight limits for all patient use equipment in clinical areas, and to have appropriate equipment available to care for obese patients. With the growing population of obese patients, hospitals must proactively purchase or rent appropriately sized equipment across the continuum.

Attaching stickers with weight limits to all equipment is one way to visually remind staff. Knowing weight limits applies to all care areas, from the emergency room, to the OR, to the ICU, to the diagnostic suites (ie, angiography, CT, MRI), to the clinics. When considering equipment weight limits, it is also important to factor in the weight of additional equipment that a patient requires such as IV pumps, monitors, and oxygen tanks. In addition, extra weight allowance in the event of cardiopulmonary resuscitation (CPR) - with additional weight from staff performing CPR - should be included.

Transfer equipment and beds are often the first necessary equipment required when an obese patient is admitted via the emergency room to the critical care area. Gurneys, wheelchairs, and beds need to be appropriately sized, and have adequate weight limits to support a patient's weight. Beds that are wide enough to adequately turn the patient side-to-side are necessary to prevent skin breakdown.[60] Recliner-type "big boy" beds limit the ability to re-position obese patients, and they often make transition to rehab difficult. Patients who work with physical therapy to transition to discharge must be able to exit from the side of their bed as they would at home. Utilizing an overhead trapeze encourages bed mobility in patients who are able to re-position themselves independently. Bariatric bedside commodes and walkers or bariatric bedpans should be used for maintaining toileting programs and promoting continence in obese patients. If a patient is incontinent, appropriate sized incontinence briefs and/or pads are required to wick away moisture and maintain skin integrity.

Lift equipment for transferring or turning obese patients is essential. Etiology of staff injury has shown that the majority of injuries are caused by repetitive movements over time.[61] Overhead ceiling lifts or free-standing lifts should be readily available for staff use.

Best practice in safe patient handling has been implemented in many care areas, and state regulations now are mandating "no lift" policies for patient care providers.[61,62] To reduce staff injury and promote patient safety, many hospitals are using specially trained roving lift teams to turn and mobilize patients. These teams often work with physical therapy to receive training on body mechanics and proper lifting technique to avoid injury.

Post-Hospitalization Planning

There is an increased incidence of discharge to nursing home post-discharge for obese patients for wound care.[7] Skilled nursing homes and rehabilitation centers often have limits on number of obese patients that they can admit due to staffing, equipment, and reimbursement restrictions.[63] Coordination of discharge planning should begin soon after admission to the ICU to prevent delays in transfer or placement.

SUMMARY

Data on skin care of critically ill obese patients is rare. Studies that assess risk factors for patients of normal weight may not apply to this patient population. Based on recommendations for normal weight patients, the following guidelines can be used until further research on the critically ill obese patient is completed.

GENERAL TREATMENT GUIDELINES FOR PREVENTING SKIN BREAKDOWN

- Use a validated pressure ulcer risk assessment tool such as the Braden scale to assess patient risk for pressure ulcer development. Assess on admission to ICU, and with any changes in patient condition.
- Prevention and treatment plans should be evidence-based and tailored to an individual's needs, taking into account patient preference and cost-effectiveness
- Treat any underlying conditions that may contribute to hypoperfusion, hypoxia, hypotension, or hyperglycemia
- Assess nutrition and feed early to prevent catabolism and malnutrition
- Perform perineal care with each episode of incontinence
- Apply barrier creams to all moist areas. (Products with ingredients: zinc oxide, dimethicone, or petrolatum)
- Patients at risk for pressure ulcer development should be placed on pressure reduction surfaces appropriate for their size
- Enhance early mobility using appropriately-sized equipment and adequate staffing
- Encourage independent bed mobility using assistive devices such as overhead trapeze and bedrails
- Decrease friction and shear using lift equipment and anti-shear sheets
- Carefully inspect all skin folds daily
- Develop interdisciplinary protocols to care for obese patients across the care continuum
- Work with supply chain managers to order appropriately-sized beds, linens, and patient-care equipment
- Work with clinical engineering to obtain correct diagnostic equipment (long and/or wide blood pressure cuffs, extra long instruments and needles, wide tracheostomy ties)
- Begin discharge planning on admission to prevent unnecessary delays in discharge and to facilitate transition to rehabilitation

REFERENCES

1. World Health Organization. Obesity and overweight fact sheet #311. Available at: http://www.who.int/mediacentre/factsheets/fs311/en/index.html. Accessed February 10, 2009.
2. Ogden CL, Carroll MD, Curtin LR, et al. Prevalence of overweight and obesity in the United States, 1999–2004. JAMA 2006;295(13):1549–55.
3. Ogden CL, Yanovski SZ, Carroll MD, et al. The epidemiology of obesity. Gastroenterology 2007;132(6):2087–102.
4. Ogden CL. Disparities in obesity prevalence in the United States: black women at risk. Am J Clin Nutr 2009;89(4):1001–2.
5. Oliveros H, Villamor E. Obesity and mortality in critically ill adults: a systematic review and meta-analysis. Obesity (Silver Spring) 2008;16(3):515–21.
6. Akinnusi ME, Pineda LA, El Solh AA. Effect of obesity on intensive care morbidity and mortality: a meta-analysis. Crit Care Med 2008;36(1):151–8.
7. Bearden DT, Rodvold KA. Dosage adjustments for antibacterials in obese patients: applying clinical pharmacokinetics. Clin Pharm 2000; 38(5):415–26.
8. Risica PM, Weinstock MA, Rakowski W, et al. Body satisfaction effect on thorough skin self-examination. Am J Prev Med 2008;35(1):68–72.
9. Garcia Hidalgo L. Dermatological complications of obesity. Am J Clin Dermatol 2002;3(7):497–506.
10. Centers for Disease Control and Prevention. National diabetes fact sheet: general information and national estimates on diabetes in the United States, 2007. Atlanta, (GA): U.S. Department of Health and Human Services, Centers for Disease Control and Prevention, 2008. Available at: http://www.cdc.gov/diabetes/pubs/pdf/ndfs_2007.pdf. Accessed February 10, 2009.
11. Jeffcoate WJ. The incidence of amputation in diabetes. Acta Chir Belg 2005; 105(2):140–4.
12. Scheinfeld NS. Obesity and dermatology. Clin Dermatol 2004;22(4):303–9.
13. Hospital Stays among Patients with Diabetes. 2004. Available at: http://www.hcup-us.ahrq.gov/reports/statbriefs/sb17.pdf. Accessed February 10, 2009.
14. Pinsolle V, Grinfeder C, Mathoulin-Pelissier S, et al. Complications analysis of 266 immediate breast reconstructions. J Plast Reconstr Aesthet Surg 2006;59(10): 1017–24.
15. Saffle JR, Morris SE, Edelman L. Fournier's gangrene: management at a regional burn center. J Burn Care Res 2008;29(1):196–203.
16. Penington AJ, Morrison WA. Skin graft failure is predicted by waist-hip ratio: a marker for metabolic syndrome. ANZ J Surg 2007;77(3):118–20.
17. Jeffcoate WJ, Chipchase SY, Ince P, et al. Assessing the outcome of the management of diabetic foot ulcers using ulcer-related and person-related measures. Diabetes Care 2006;29(8):1784–7.
18. Danielsson G, Eklof B, Grandinetti A, et al. The influence of obesity on chronic venous disease. Vasc Endovascular Surg 2002;36(4):271–6.
19. Peterson M, Schwab W, McCutcheon K, et al. Effects of elevating the head of bed on interface pressure in volunteers. Crit Care Med 2008;36(11):3038–42.
20. Frankenfield DC, Coleman A, Alam S, et al. Analysis of estimation methods for resting metabolic rate in critically ill adults. JPEN J Parenter Enteral Nutr 2009; 33(1):27–36.
21. Janniger CK, Schwartz RA, Szepietowski JC, et al. Intertrigo and common secondary skin infections. Am Fam Physician 2005;72(5):833–8.

22. Sommer DM, Jenisch S, Suchan M, et al. Increased prevalence of the metabolic syndrome in patients with moderate to severe psoriasis. Arch Dermatol Res 2006; 298(7):321–8.
23. Setty AR, Curhan G, Choi HK. Obesity, waist circumference, weight change, and the risk of psoriasis in women: Nurses' Health Study II. Arch Intern Med 2007; 167(15):1670–5.
24. Gisondi P, Tessari G, Conti A, et al. Prevalence of metabolic syndrome in patients with psoriasis: a hospital-based case-control study. Br J Dermatol 2007;157(1): 68–73.
25. Johnston A, Arnadottir S, Gudjonsson JE, et al. Obesity in psoriasis: leptin and resistin as mediators of cutaneous inflammation. Br J Dermatol 2008;159(2): 342–50.
26. Kourosh AS, Miner A, Menter A. Psoriasis as the marker of underlying systemic disease. Skin Therapy Lett 2008;13(1):1–5.
27. Pressure ulcers in America: prevalence, incidence, and implications for the future. An executive summary of the National Pressure Ulcer Advisory Panel monograph. Adv Skin Wound Care 2001;14(4):208–15.
28. Braden BJ, Bergstrom N. Clinical utility of the Braden scale for Predicting Pressure Sore Risk. Decubitus 1989;2(3):44–6 50-1.
29. Black J, Baharestani MM, Cuddigan J, et al. National Pressure Ulcer Advisory Panel's updated pressure ulcer staging system. Adv Skin Wound Care 2007; 20(5):269–74.
30. Kraemer-Aguiar LG, Laflor CM, Bouskela E. Skin microcirculatory dysfunction is already present in normoglycemic subjects with metabolic syndrome. Metabolism 2008;57(12):1740–6.
31. Wound, Ostomy, and Continence Nurses Society (WOCN). Guideline for prevention and management of pressure ulcers, Glenview (IL): Wound, Ostomy, and Continence Nurses Society (WOCN); (WOCN clinical practice guideline; no. 2) 2003. p. 52.
32. Stechmiller JK, Cowan L, Whitney JD, et al. Guidelines for the prevention of pressure ulcers. Wound Repair Regen 2008;16(2):151–68.
33. National Pressure Ulcer Advisory Panel (NPUAP). Advances in skin and wound care. Pressure ulcer prevalence, cost and risk assessment: consensus development conference statement—The National Pressure Ulcer Advisory Panel. Decubitus 1989;(2):24–8.
34. Elsner JJ, Gefen A. Is obesity a risk factor for deep tissue injury in patients with spinal cord injury? J Biomech 2008;41(16):3322–31.
35. Dibsie LG. Implementing evidence-based practice to prevent skin breakdown. Crit Care Nurs Q 2008;31(2):140–9.
36. Baldelli P, Paciella M. Creation and implementation of a pressure ulcer prevention bundle improves patient outcomes. Am J Med Qual 2008;23(2):136–42.
37. de Laat EH, Pickkers P, Schoonhoven L, et al. Guideline implementation results in a decrease of pressure ulcer incidence in critically ill patients. Crit Care Med 2007;35(3):815–20.
38. Robinson C, Gloekner M, Bush S, et al. Determining the efficacy of a pressure ulcer prevention program by collecting prevalence and incidence data: a unit-based effort. Ostomy Wound Manage 2003;49(5):44–6, 48–51.
39. Tablan OC, Anderson LJ, Besser R, et al. Guidelines for preventing health-care–associated pneumonia, 2003: recommendations of CDC and the Healthcare Infection Control Practices Advisory Committee. MMWR Recomm Rep 2004; 53(RR-3):1–36.

40. Elamin EM, Camporesi E. Evidence-based nutritional support in the intensive care unit. Int Anesthesiol Clin 2009;47(1):121–38.
41. Arthurs ZM, Cuadrado D, Sohn V, et al. Post-bariatric panniculectomy: pre-panniculectomy body mass index impacts the complication profile. Am J Surg 2007;193(5):567–70 [discussion: 570].
42. Bostanjian D, Anthone GJ, Hamoui N, et al. Rhabdomyolysis of gluteal muscles leading to renal failure: a potentially fatal complication of surgery in the morbidly obese. Obes Surg 2003;13(2):302–5.
43. Shibutani K, Inchiosa MA Jr, Sawada K, et al. Accuracy of pharmacokinetic models for predicting plasma fentanyl concentrations in lean and obese surgical patients: derivation of dosing weight ("pharmacokinetic mass"). Anesthesiology 2004;101(3):603–13.
44. Lemmens HJ, Brodsky JB. Anesthetic drugs and bariatric surgery. Expert Rev Neurother 2006;6(7):1107–13.
45. Truog RD, Campbell ML, Curtis JR, et al. Recommendations for end-of-life care in the intensive care unit: a consensus statement by the American College [corrected] of Critical Care Medicine. Crit Care Med 2008;36(3): 953–63.
46. Wall PD, Deucy EE, Glantz JC, et al. Vertical skin incisions and wound complications in the obese parturient. Obstet Gynecol 2003;102(5 Pt 1):952–6.
47. Hahler B. Surgical wound dehiscence. Medsurg Nurs 2006;15(5):296–300 [quiz 301].
48. Shermak MA, Rotellini-Coltvet LA, Chang D. Seroma development following body contouring surgery for massive weight loss: patient risk factors and treatment strategies. Plast Reconstr Surg 2008;122(1):280–8.
49. Nemerofsky RB, Oliak DA, Capella JF. Body lift: an account of 200 consecutive cases in the massive weight loss patient. Plast Reconstr Surg 2006;117(2): 414–30.
50. Lazarus GS, Cooper DM, Knighton DR, et al. Definitions and guidelines for assessment of wounds and evaluation of healing. Arch Dermatol 1994;130(4): 489–93.
51. Wound, Ostomy, and Continence Nurses Society (WOCN). Guideline for management of wounds in patients with lower-extremity neuropathic disease. Glenview (IL): Wound, Ostomy, and Continence Nurses Society (WOCN); (WOCN clinical practice guideline; no. 3) 2004. p. 57.
52. Wound, Ostomy, and Continence Nurses Society (WOCN). Guideline for management of wounds in patients with lower-extremity neuropathic disease. Glenview (IL): Wound, Ostomy, and Continence Nurses Society (WOCN); (WOCN clinical practice guideline; no. 4) 2005. p. 42.
53. Bergstrom N, Bennett MA, Carlson CE, et al. Pressure ulcer treatment clinical practice guideline. Quick Reference Guide for Clinicians, no. 15. Rockville, (MD): U.S. Department of Health and Human Services, Public Health Service, Agency for Health Care Policy and Research (AHCPR) Pub. No. 95-0653. 1994.
54. Cheymol G. Effects of obesity on pharmacokinetics implications for drug therapy. Clin Pharm 2000;39(3):215–31.
55. Langemo DK. When the goal is palliative care. Adv Skin Wound Care 2006;19(3): 148–54.
56. Naylor WA. A guide to wound managment in palliative care. Int J Palliat Nurs 2005;11(11):572, 574–9 [discussion: 579].

57. Hodgin KE, Nordon-Craft A, McFann KK, et al. Physical therapy utilization in intensive care units: results from a national survey. Crit Care Med 2009;37(2): 561–6 [quiz 566–8].
58. Gallagher S, Arzouman J, Lacovara J, et al. Criteria-based protocols and the obese patient: planning care for a high-risk population. Ostomy Wound Manage 2004;50(5):32–4, 36, 38 passim.
59. Gallagher S, Langlois C, Spacht DW, et al. Preplanning with protocols for skin and wound care in obese patients. Adv Skin Wound Care 2004;17(8):436–41 [quiz 442–3].
60. Kramer KL. WOC nurses as advocates for patients who are morbidly obese: a case study promoting the use of bariatric beds. J Wound Ostomy Continence Nurs 2004;31(6):379–84 [discussion: 384–7].
61. Nelson A, Baptiste AS. Evidence-based practices for safe patient handling and movement. Orthop Nurs 2006;25(6):366–79.
62. de Castro AB, Hagan P, Nelson A. Prioritizing safe patient handling: The American Nurses Association's Handle With Care Campaign. J Nurs Adm 2006; 36(7–8):363–9.
63. Bradway C, DiResta J, Fleshner I, et al. Obesity in nursing homes: a critical review. J Am Geriatr Soc 2008;56(8):1528–35.

Pain Management in Critically Ill Obese Patients

Sonia M. Astle, RN, MS

KEYWORDS

• Pain management • Morbid obesity • Bariatrics
• Analgesics • Pain pathways

Achieving pain control in critically ill patients is a challenging problem, generally, for the health care team and becomes even more challenging in regard to the morbidly obese patient. Obese patients may experience drug malabsorption and distribution, leading to either subtherapeutic or toxic drug levels. To manage pain effectively for the critically ill obese patient, nurses must have an understanding of how obesity alters a patient's physiologic response to injury and illness. In addition, nurses must be knowledgeable about physiologic mechanisms, types and manifestations of pain, differing patterns of drug absorption and distribution, pharmacokinetic properties of analgesic medications, and pain management strategies.

The prevalence of morbid obesity is escalating in the United States and morbid obesity is a major public health concern worldwide. Recent data demonstrate that 32% of adults in the United States are obese with a body mass index (BMI) greater than 30 kg/m^2 and nearly 5% or about nine million people are considered morbidly obese, correlating with at a BMI of greater than 40 kg/m^2.[1] There is a strong association between obesity and chronic medical conditions including: cardiovascular disease, hypertension, type II diabetes, hyperlipidemia, arthritis, debilitating pulmonary conditions, and certain types of cancer.[2] In a recent study in a family practice outpatient setting, a BMI greater than 35 kg/m^2 was a risk factor for elevated pain scores that correlated positively to abdominal, back, extremity, joint and muscle pain, leg pain when walking, and headaches.[3] The incidence of morbidly obese patients with a critical illness is approximately 14 cases per 1000 nonsurgical ICU admissions per year.[4] Annual bariatric procedures in the United States have risen from 12,775 cases in 1997 to 70,000 in 2002 to over 103,000 in 2008 and are estimated to become 250,000 cases by 2010.[5–7] The direct cost in caring for obese patients represents 5.7% of the national health expenditure in the United States.[8] Although obesity in critical illness has not been found to impact mortality, it does prolong the duration of mechanical ventilation and prolonged intensive care unit (ICU)

Department of Critical Care, Inova Fairfax Hospital, 3300 Gallows Road, Falls Church, VA 22042, USA
E-mail address: Sonia.astle@inova.org

Crit Care Nurs Clin N Am 21 (2009) 323–339
doi:10.1016/j.ccell.2009.07.012
0899-5885/09/$ – see front matter © 2009 Elsevier Inc. All rights reserved.

length-of-stay.[9] With the increasing prevalence of obesity and bariatric procedures, morbidly obese patients requiring intensive care treatment is proliferating.

Pain control, in itself, is associated with significant increases in health care costs, through extended lengths of hospital stay and an increase in hospital readmissions.[10] Uncontrolled pain delays wound healing, contributes to muscle deconditioning, and increases complications associated with critical illness, while causing additional physical, psychological and emotional distress.[11] The benefits of achieving optimal pain management facilitate early mobilization preventing thromboembolic and pulmonary complications, and sleep disruption while enhancing patients' health-related quality of life.[12–14]

PATHOPHYSIOLOGY OF PAIN

Regardless of a patient's body size, pain is an unpleasant subjective sensation resulting from a physiologic response to a variety of noxious mechanical, thermal or chemical stimuli and is associated with physical, psychological and emotional distress.[11,15,16] The mechanisms that contribute to pain are not completely understood. Researchers are beginning to focus on the complexity of pain perception and believe that an individual's perception of pain includes cellular, molecular, genetic, psychological and cultural factors.[16,17] Other influencing factors include: gender, age, past experiences, ethnicity, and temperament; these factors impact the perception of an individual's pain.[18–20]

Several theories attempt to explain the mechanism of pain. Recent theories include the "gate control" and neuromatrix mechanisms. The gate control theory, first presented by Malzack and Wall, describes the brain as the active system for filtering, selecting and modulating sensory information.[21] The brain is the "gate keeper" and is able to increase or decrease the flow of pain impulses from peripheral nerves. During further research by Malzack, the gate theory evolved into the neuromatrix theory of pain that describes a genetic uniqueness for every person.[22] Multiple factors contribute to each person's pain experience including sensory, visual, and emotional inputs and one's cognitive interpretation of these factors. Every individual has a different network of neurons, referred to as the neuromatrix, and therefore experiences pain differently than anyone else.

A review of pain physiology is helpful in understanding the way analgesics work. Nociceptors are nerve endings that respond to pain. Nociceptive pain is the perception and transmission of painful stimuli and it occurs when nerve endings in the periphery are activated by a noxious stimulus such as tissue damage. After being activated, neurotransmitters, including norepinephrine, dopamine, serotonin and gamma aminobutyric acid (GABA), allow the pain message to ascend through the dorsal horn of the spinal cord to the brainstem by way of the anterolateral tract and enter the thalamus where perception about the location and intensity of the pain occurs. The thalamus relays the pain stimulus to the to the autonomic system increasing heart rate and blood pressure and to the emotional (limbic system) and memory centers of the brain that may trigger fear and impact the individual's current emotional status (**Fig. 1**).[23]

Tissue damage activates nociceptors and the pain process begins. A local inflammatory response is sustained with the release of various chemical mediators including histamine, substance P, bradykinin, and prostaglandins. These mediators cause endothelial vasodilation, vasoconstriction or vascular permeability; they sensitize functional nociceptors and activate those that have been dormant, causing the pain to amplify.[14,24,25] Two types of nociceptive nerve fibers transmit the pain stimulus from visceral and somatic areas to the brain: A-delta fibers are myelinated and allow

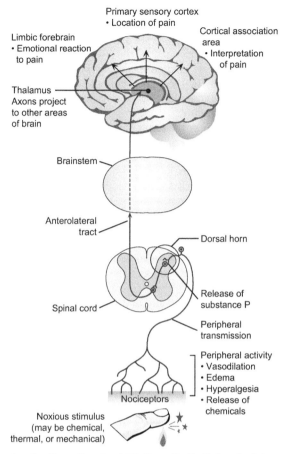

Fig. 1. Pathways of pain. *From* Copstead LE, Banasik JL. Pathophysiology. St. Louis (MO): Elsevier Saunders; 2005; with permission.

a very rapid transmission of the pain sensation, often causing the body's reflex to occur before the pain is felt. The sensation of pain from A-delta fibers is sharp and quickly dissipates. C fibers are unmyelinated and transmit the pain signal much more slowly than the A-delta fibers. Pain transmitted slowly through C fibers is felt constantly as a dull, burning or aching sensation.

TYPES OF PAIN

Patients experience different types of pain that are either acute, chronic or neuropathic in nature. Acute pain is limited in time but can progress to chronic pain if not adequately treated.[14,15] Acute pain is usually nocioceptive in nature and includes somatic, visceral, and referred pain. Somatic pain occurs at the tissue level, either superficial, involving the skin and subcutaneous tissue or deep, involving the musculoskeletal tissue. It can be characterized as sharp, burning, dull, aching or cramping, and is usually well localized. Examples of somatic pain include incisional pain, muscle spasms, and the pain that occurs with bone metastasis. Visceral pain refers to pain in the organs and linings of body cavities. This pain may be caused by procedural pain associated with chest tube insertion, bladder distension or infiltrates into organs such as pancreatic cancer. This pain is diffuse, cramping, sharp or stabbing, and is poorly localized. Referred pain often occurs with visceral pain and is felt at a location other than the site of injury. This phenomenon is thought to occur because the area of injury and the area that senses the pain are supplied by nerves in the same spinal segment. An example of referred pain is myocardial pain that is felt in the jaw or shoulder but not in the chest.

Opioid analgesics are the cornerstone of pharmacologic treatment for acute pain management. Two analgesic agents acting by different mechanisms via the same route are often more effective than using only one analgesic.[12,26] For example, epidural opioids in combination with a local epidural anesthetic or intravenous opioids in combination with ketorolac are proving to provide superior analgesic management. In the obese population, epidural local anesthetics and/or narcotics and intrathecal narcotics have been shown to be a safe and effective form of postoperative analgesia following bariatric surgical procedures.[26,27] Preemptive pain management (ie, providing analgesia before pain begins or immediately after the patient experiences pain) is key in preventing chronic pain syndromes.

Acute pain can become chronic pain due to persistent stimulation of the unmyelinated C nerves fibers. Constant nerve stimulations cause the release of excitatory amino acids and is explained by a phenomenon known as windup.[25] During constant nerve firing, there is a progressive buildup of electrical response in the central nervous system (CNS), nerve transmission becomes faster and faster. Constant stimulation of nerve fibers over time causes nerves to change, a process called neuroplasty. Neuroplasty leads to an increase in the intensity, duration, and distribution of the pain. Even if the original injury completely heals, the neuroplastic affects causes pain to continue.[14,25]

Neuropathic pain is a complex form of chronic pain that is caused by injury of peripheral nerves rather than stimulation of nociceptors.[25] Peripheral and central sensitization, which is an increase in the sensitivity of spinal neurons, develop as damaged nerves become abnormally excited. Patients experiencing neuropathic pain feel numbness, tenderness or a burning, stabbing, or shooting sensation. A complete neurologic examination is essential to evaluate sensory, motor, cranial nerve, reflex, cerebellar, cognitive, and emotional function. Sensory evaluation may elicit the presence of hyperalgesia (an increased sensitivity to pain), or allodynia (pain caused by benign stimuli such as touch). These findings are significant symptoms that accompany neuropathic pain, especially when no apparent skin pathology is present. Chronic pain requires multimodal pharmacologic treatment including tricyclic antidepressants that work by inhibiting the reuptake of neurotransmitters in the dorsal horn, anticonvulsants to decrease the excitatory nerve pathways, and local anesthetics to block nerve transmission.

PAIN ASSESSMENT IN THE CRITICALLY ILL PATIENT

Appropriate assessment and management of pain is essential for optimal patient outcomes. Evidenced-based guidelines and position statements guide many professional health care specialties and decrease inconsistencies in pain assessment and variations in practice. Critically ill patients are often not able to communicate their discomfort because of mechanical intubation, sedation, or being in a state of unconsciousness and they are at greater risk for inadequate analgesia. In 2006, the American Society for Pain Management Nursing published a position statement and five clinical practice recommendations for pain assessment in the nonverbal patient (**Table 1**).[28] Assessing the patient's pain through self-report should be the first line for pain assessment to determine the patient's ability to communicate. Self-report in

Table 1	
Guiding principles and recommendations for pain assessment in the unconscious patient	
Guiding Principle	**Limitations**
Self-report: requires serial assessments	Delirium, endotracheal tubes, decreased level of consciousness, sedatives
Identify potential causes of pain or discomfort	Practitioner must predict sources of pain (eg, injuries, invasive procedures, wound care, suctioning, repositioning, immobility)
Observation of patient behavior	Use is not appropriate with paralytic agents or individuals who are paralyzed or have neurologic diseases limiting physical responses
Surrogate reporting of pain	Caregivers/family members assessment of the patient's pain may be inaccurate
Analgesic trial: escalating doses of analgesic medication	Given if pain is suspected, subjective assessment

Data from Herr K, Coyne PJ, Manworren R, et al. Pain assessment in the nonverbal patient: position statement with clinical practice recommendations. Pain Manag Nurs 2006;7(2):49; and Puntillo KA, White C, Morris AB, et al. Patients' perceptions and responses to procedural pain: results from Thunder Project II. Am J of Crit Care 2001;10(4):238–51.

this population has many limitations, however. Mechanical ventilation, sedation, cognitive impairment, or delirium may hamper the nurse's ability to obtain a reliable pain assessment. Potential causes of pain in critically ill patients are also a focus of these recommendations; the nurse must be vigilant to assess for pain during routine procedures such as suctioning, repositioning, dressing changes, and pain caused by immobility.[28,29] Oversedation may mask the patient's underlying pain (**Table 2**).[30]

Observing the patient's behavior has been the traditional method nurses use to assess pain in nonverbal patients. Two frequently employed behavioral assessment tools include the Behavioral Pain Scale (**Table 3**)[31] and the Critical-Care Pain Observational Tool (**Table 4**).[32] These scales have been tested in the nonverbal adult population and are helpful assessment tools, however, they are not beneficial for patients who are pharmacologically or otherwise paralyzed, oversedated, or who have underlying diseases such as myasthenia gravis, Guillain-Barre syndrome, or critical illness polyneuropathy. Patients falling into this category cannot demonstrate the behavioral cues such as facial grimacing and hand clenching needed for pain scoring. Research does not support using vital signs as a sole indicator of either pain or the absence of pain.[33]

The health care team should also rely on surrogate reporting of the patient's pain by family members and caregivers. These individuals can frequently supply additional information relating to the patient's responses to pain and treatment modalities that have previously been effective to relieve pain. If pain is suspected but unable to be measured, an analgesic trial should be initiated.[28] During this trial the analgesic medication is slowly titrated upward, frequent assessments are needed to evaluate the patient's response.

FACTORS AFFECTING PHARMACOKINETICS IN OBESE INDIVIDUALS

Obesity is a chronic disease characterized by multiple physiologic changes. Adipose tissue is the common denominator in a triad of characteristics including inflammation,

Table 2
Harmful effects of constant pain

Cardiovascular	Increased heart rate, blood pressure, cardiac output, systemic vascular resistance and myocardial oxygenation, hypercoagulation, deep vein thromboses
Respiratory	Decrease flow of oxygen, pulmonary shunting, hypoxia, atelectasis, pneumonia, infection
Gastrointestinal	Decreased gastric and bowel motility
Musculoskeletal	Muscle spasm, fatigue, immobility
Cognitive	Confusion, reduced cognitive function
Endocrine	Increased adrenocorticotropic hormone, cortisol, antidiuretic hormone, aldosterone, renin, epinephrine, norepinephrine, interlukin 1, growth hormone, glucagon, decreased insulin and testosterone
Metabolic	Gluconeogenesis, hepatic glycogenolysis, hyperglycemia, glucose intolerance, insulin resistance, muscle protein catabolism, increased lipolysis
Genitourinary	Decreased urinary output, urinary retention, hypokalemia
Quality of life	Sleeplessness, anxiety, fear, hopelessness, increased thoughts of suicide

Data from McCaffery M, Pasero C. Assessment: underlying complexities, misconceptions, and practical tools. In: Pain Clinical Manual. St. Louis (MO): Mosby; 1999.

hypercoagulability and insulin resistance. This pathology is common in obese patients experiencing critical illness. Adipose tissue serves as an energy reservoir for excess fat accumulation. The pathophysiology of excess fat stores begins by a change in the cell's normal structure. Cells become larger in diameter and fat deposits interfere with structures around the cell such as nerves and blood vessels and affect the mechanics of virtually every body system. Adipose tissue has been found to be

Table 3
Behavioral pain score for sedated patients

Item	Description	Score
Facial expression	Relaxed	1
	Partially tightened (eg, brow lowering)	2
	Fully tightened (eg, eyelid closing)	3
	Grimacing	4
Upper limbs	No movement	1
	Partially bent	2
	Fully bent with finger flexion	3
	Permanently retracted	4
Compliance with ventilation	Tolerating movement	1
	Coughing but tolerating ventilation for most of the time	2
	Fighting ventilator	3
	Unable to control ventilation	4
Total, range		3–12

From Payen J, Bru, O, Bosson J, et al. Assessing pain in critically ill sedated patients by using a behavioral pain scale. Critical Care Medicine 2001;29(12):2259. Lippincott Williams & Wilkins; with permission.

Table 4			
Critical care pain observation tool (CPOT)			
Indicator	Description	Score	
Facial expression	No muscular tension, observed	Relaxed, neutral	0
	Presence of frowning, brow lowering, orbit tightening, and levator contraction	Tense	1
	All of the above facial movements plus eyelid tightly closed	Grimacing	2
Body movements	Does not move at all (does not necessarily mean absence of pain)	Absence of movements	0
	Slow, cautious movements, touching or rubbing the pain site, seeking attention through movements	Protection	1
	Pulling tube, attempting to sit up, moving limbs/thrashing, not following commands, striking at staff, trying to climb out of bed	Restlessness	2
Muscle tension	No resistance to passive movements	Relaxed	0
	Resistance to passive movements	Tense, rigid	1
	Strong resistance to passive movements, inability to complete them	Very tense or rigid	2
Compliance with the ventilator (intubated patients)	Alarms not activated, easy ventilation	Tolerating ventilator or movement	0
	Alarms stop spontaneously	Coughing but tolerating	1
	Asynchrony; blocking ventilation, alarms frequently activated	Fighting ventilator	2
OR vocalization (extubated patients)	Talking in normal tone or no sound	Talking in normal tone or no sound	0
	Sighing, moaning	Sighing, moaning	1
	Crying out, sobbing	Crying out, sobbing	2
Total, range		0–8	

From Gelinas C, Fillion L, Puntillo KA, et al. Validation of the critical-care pain observation tool in adult patients. American Journal of Critical Care 2006;15(4):421; with permission.

a rich source of tumor necrosis factor alpha and interliukin-6. Both are cytokines produced primarily by monocytes and macrophages and help to regulate the immune system by causing cellular apoptosis and inflammation. In addition, obese individuals have increased concentrations of fibrinogen and plasminogen activator inhibitor-1 and lower concentrations of antithrombin-III, leading to decreased fibrinolysis and a constant state of hypercoagualabily.[34] Excessive weight affects every organ system in the body.

The cardiovascular effects of obesity significantly relate to drug absorption. Approximately 3 mL of blood volume are required to perfuse 100 g of adipose tissue, so blood volume increases directly with body weight.[35] The expanded blood volume requirements to adipose tissue increase cardiac output and myocardial workload resulting in ventricular dilatation and hypertrophy, congestive heart failure, acute myocardial ischemia, and dysrhythmias. Obese patients therefore may not tolerate large volumes of fluid during resuscitation and require close monitoring to prevent cardiac ischemia and pulmonary edema.

There is a large amount of adipose tissue in the pharynx of the obese patient that may present difficulty when managing the airway. Additional adipose tissue impedes the ability to intubate the patient and poses a potential risk of airway obstruction after the patient is extubated.[36–38] The obese patient is at risk of resedation, a phenomenon that occurs when there is a redistribution of lipophilic anesthetics or analgesic agents from the adipose tissue to the bloodstream.[36]

The term "metabolic x syndrome" has been coined to refer to a group of cardiac risk factors associated with obesity. Insulin resistance, hyperinsulinemia, hyperglycemia, coronary artery disease, hypertension and hyperlipidemia are common comorbidities of excess adipose tissue.[39] As excess fat stores accumulate, the pancreas secretes more insulin causing lipid mobilization to slow and the breakdown of protein to accelerate.

The effect of protein breakdown causes a high fat-to-muscle ratio and affects the amount of water available for drug absorption.

PHARMACOKINETIC FACTORS ASSOCIATED WITH OBESITY

Few pharmacokinetic studies guide medication administration for obese patients and among those completed, antibiotics and sedatives have been the predominate focus. Finding the optimal therapeutic medication dose in obese patients is of concern so that sub- and supratherapeutic doses are not given.

The main factors affecting tissue distribution of drugs include the affinity of the drug for plasma proteins, body composition and regional circulation.[40,41] Normal blood distribution includes 5% blood flow to adipose tissue, 73% to the viscera, and 22% to lean tissue.[42,43] Obese patients have both more lean body mass as well as fat mass than do non-obese patients; however, the percentage of fat per kg of body weight is increased with obesity. This ratio of lean-to-fat body mass alters blood distribution; there is less blood flow to the adipose tissue but organs in obese patients remain relatively well perfused as long as there are no confounding medical conditions. Because muscle tissue holds more water than adipose tissue, medications that are hydrophilic in nature may not be distributed evenly through adipose tissue. Hydrophilic drugs therefore should be initially based on ideal body weight (IBW). Lipophilic drugs are well absorbed by adipose tissue, so the dose necessary to gain effect should be based on the patient's actual body weight (ABW); however, because of the circulation pattern to adipose tissue, the elimination half-life may increase, prolonging the effect of the drug. Researchers have found a correctional factor to ABW may be needed to determine the "pharmacokinetic mass" when determining the dose of some lipophilic drugs.[44] Renal function also must be a factor to analyze when determining drug dosing.[45]

Patients with normal renal function will have an increase in drug clearance; however, comorbidities associated with obesity, such as hypertension and diabetes often cause a decrease in renal function.[46] The Cockcroft-Gault equation is commonly used to predict glomerular filtration rate (GFR) but uses only IBW. The disparity between lean and adipose tissue in obese individuals may lead to overestimation or underestimation of GFR when using this formula. The Salazar-Corcoran equation has been found to better predict GFR by using multiple factors including gender, actual weight, age, and height and serum creatinine (**Box 1**).[47]

CLINICAL PHARMACOLOGY OF OPIOIDS

Opioids are naturally occurring alkaloids that have been used to manage pain throughout history. The first record of cultivating the poppy to produce opium dates

---

Box 1
Salazar-Corcoran equation for creatinine clearance

$$(Male)ClCr = \frac{(137 - age) \times \left[(0.285 \times Wt) + (12.1 \times Ht^2)\right]}{(51 \times SCr)}$$

$$(Female)ClCr = \frac{(146 - age) \times \left[(0.287 \times Wt) + (9.74 \times Ht^2)\right]}{(60 \times SCr)}$$

Wt, actual body weight in kg; Ht, height in meters.

From Salazar DE, Corcoran GB. Predicting creatinine clearance and renal drug clearance in obese patients from estimated fat-free body mass. Am J Med 1988;84:1053–60.

---

back to 3400 BC in Mesopotamia. The term "opioid" describes all medications that work at opioid receptors. These receptors are found within the central nervous system and in the peripheral tissues and are normally stimulated by endogenous peptides such as endorphins that are produced in response to tissue injury and other noxious stimuli. The three major opioid receptors, Mu, Kappa and Delta, are controlled by different genes and have been named with Greek letters based on their prototype agonists.[48,49]

Most opioids prescribed for clinical analgesia create their effect by stimulating the morphine or Mu (μ) receptors so they are referred to as mu agonists. Morphine, hydromorphone, and fentanyl are examples of pure opioid agonists, therefore they are the most potent analgesics. Mu receptors are often called "morphine opioid receptors" (MOR). They are found in the brainstem and thalamus and have been subdivided into Mu1 and Mu2 receptors. Mu1 receptors associate with analgesia, euphoria and serenity and Mu2 with respiratory depression, pruritus, prolacatin release, dependence, anorexia and sedation.[48] The other important Mu receptors are Kappa and Delta receptors.

Kappa (κ) receptors or kappa opioid receptors (KOR) are responsible for sedation, dyspnea, dependence, dysphoria, respiratory depression, and spinal analgesia. They are found in the limbic area, the brainstem, and spinal cord. The agonist for kappa receptors is ketocyclazocine. Delta (δ) receptors are located in the brain and are thought to be responsible for psychomimetic and dysphoric effects. The agonist for delta receptors is delta-alanine-delta-leucine-enkephalin.[49] The differences in the opioid agonists (or medications) are based on their varying effect on these three receptors sites.

Opioids are classified by their medial use and level of addition (Schedule I–V) and by their actions on the receptor site, affinity and efficacy (**Table 5**). Affinity measures the strength of the interaction between the drug and the receptor, while efficacy measures the activity of the drug at the receptor. Both the affinity and efficacy of a drug determine its action. Strong agonists have both a high affinity and efficacy; partial agonists have a high affinity with low efficacy; and an antagonist has affinity but no efficacy. For example, a strong agonist, morphine, has both a strong affinity and efficacy; a partial or weak agonist such as codeine has a weak affinity and efficacy; while naloxone, an antagonist has affinity but no efficacy at the receptor site. When administering partial agonists, a higher dose is not equivalent to more effective analgesia. Higher doses of partial agonists usually equate to more opioid side effects.

Opioid metabolism occurs primarily in the liver where opioids transform into many different metabolites by way of the cytochrome P_{450} (CPY$_{450}$) enzyme system. Both

Table 5
Pharmacokinetic properties of selected opioids

Opioid	Schedule	Solubility	Half Life	Action on Receptor	Type of Pain
Morphine	II	Hydrophilic	2–3.5 hours	Strong agonist	Moderate to severe
Codeine	II	Hydrophilic	2.5–3 hours	Weak agonist	Mild
Hydrocodone	III	Hydrophilic	2.5–4	Strong agonist	Moderate to severe
Oxycodone	II	Hydrophilic	2–3		
Hydromorphone	II	Hydrophilic	2–3	Strong agonist	Moderate to severe
Methadone	II	Lipophilic	24 (12–150)	Strong agonist	Severe neuropathic and opioid-resistant
Fentanyl[a]	II	Lipophilic	3–4	Strong agonist	Moderate to severe

[a] Correctional factor for fentanyl dosing in the obese patient $52/(1 + [196.4 \times e^{-0.025\, ABW} - 53.66]/100)$. Pieracci FM, Barie PS, Pomp A. Critical care of the bariatric patient. Critical Care Medicine 2006;34(6):1796–803.

Data from Trescot AM, Datta S, Lee M, et al. Opioid pharmacology. Pain Physician 2008;11:S133–53.

the side effects of opioids as well as their analgesic effects are directly related to these metabolites. Many factors contribute to the rate of metabolism including gender, genetic makeup, age, diet, disease state, and concurrent use of medications.[45,49] Potentially dangerous drug interactions may also occur with concomitantly administered medications because of competitive metabolism with varying CPY_{450} isoforms in the liver.

SPECIFIC OPIOIDS
Morphine

Morphine is the prototype Mu receptor opioid and is clinically used to treat moderate to severe pain because it has both a high affinity and efficacy at the receptor site. It is a relatively long acting opioid with rare drug-to-drug interactions. Multiple side effects can be expected from morphine, however. Histamine release may cause bronchospasms, peripheral vasodilation resulting in hypotension and urticaria. Respiratory depression is frequently linked to over medication and may rapidly lead to respiratory acidosis. Morphine decreases sympathetic tone causing orthostatic hypotension, causes spasm of the biliary smooth muscle, and decreases intestinal mobility. Morphine directly stimulates chemoreceptors in the brain that may cause nausea and vomiting. Patients with sulfa allergies are at a high risk for anaphylactic reactions due to the sulfites used for parenteral preparations of morphine.

Codeine

Codeine is the prototype of the weak opioid analgesics with a potency about 50% of morphine. It is considered a "prodrug" meaning that it is inactive or relatively inactive until it is metabolized into its active metabolite. Codeine is metabolized to morphine and is highly susceptible to drug–drug interactions. Side effects of codeine are similar to other opioids and include respiratory depression, mental depression, nausea, vomiting, diarrhea, constipation, dizziness and headache, although more severe side effects including hypotension and anaphylaxis have been reported.[12] Interestingly, lower doses of codeine may cause more nausea than higher doses because of competing effects within the chemoreceptor trigger zone.[49]

Hydrocodone

Hydrocodone is the most widely used opioid and is available only in combination with other nonopioid analgesics such as ibuprofen and acetaminophen. In these combinations, hydrocodone is considered a Schedule II drug. Like codeine, hydrocodone is also considered a prodrug as it converts to hydromorphone during the metabolism process. Hydromorphone has a high affinity to the Mu receptors and therefore is prescribed for moderate to moderately severe pain. This medication is also widely used as an antitussive to control dry, painful paroxysmal coughing.

Oxycodone

Oxycodone is a semi-synthetic, Schedule II drug with a half-life of 2.5 to 3 hours and is prepared both in pure form and in combination with Tylenol (Percocet, Roxocet) or aspirin (Percodan, Roxiprin). OxyContin is the sustained release form of oxycodone. It is not considered a prodrug although it does, to some extent, metabolize to oxymorphone. Oxycodone is active at multiple receptor sites including Mu and Kappa and has both analgesic and sedation effects.

Hydromorphone

Hydromorphone (Palladone, Dilaudid) is a Schedule II, semisynthetic opioid agonist and works primarily on Mu receptors with some activity on Delta receptors. It is hydrophilic and is 7 to 11 times more potent than morphine. Hydromorphone is available in oral, intravenous, intramuscular and subcutaneous preparations. The onset of action for the oral, immediate release preparation is 30 minutes with a duration of action of 4 hours. Like all opioids, Hydromorphone is metabolized in the liver and excreted by the kidneys. It is preferred over morphine for patients with renal failure because of the toxic metabolite accumulation associated with morphine.

Fentanyl

Fentanyl is a synthetic, lipophilic opioid with a rapid onset of action and binds tightly to the Mu receptor. Fentanyl has a potency of 50–100 times that of morphine but has minimal histamine-related vasodilation. Drug distribution correlates to the amount of adipose tissue, but using the patient's ABW to calculate the effective dose may lead to supratherapeutic drug levels. For this reason, a correctional factor should be used to calculate the "pharmacokinetic mass" based on the patient's total body clearance for maintenance dosing (see **Table 5**).[50] Fentanyl is available in parenteral, intrathecal, transbuccal, intranasal, and transdermal preparations. In general, medications administered to obese patients via the transdermal route are not well absorbed because of the lower amount of blood circulation to adipose tissue, although there is little available research to support this theory. Fentanyl is the preferred analgesic for critically ill patients who are hemodynamically unstable or that display histamine related symptoms when given morphine.[51]

Methadone

Methadone is a lipophilic, synthetic opioid that is unrelated in structure to standard opioids but produces many of the same effects. Like all opioid, methadone works at the Mu receptor sites. It is used for analgesia, as an antitussive, and for maintenance of anti-addiction to other opioids. Methadone has been found to be particularly effective in managing chronic neuropathtic pain because of its long duration of action. It is administered orally and can be prepared in solution or crushed and administered via a nasogastic tube. Methadone is metabolized in the liver and the intestine and is excreted in the feces. It has no active metabolites. The lipophilic properties of methadone result in a very high drug distribution in the adipose tissues causing an extremely long duration of action with a half-life, anywhere between 12 and 150 hours.[49] This individual variability is a result of genetic factors that control the production of the enzymes needed for the drug's metabolism. The analgesic effects of methadone are shorter lasting than is the half-life of the drug, so patients who are receiving methadone for pain control usually will need multiple daily dosing as opposed to the daily dosing regimen prescribed to control opioid addiction. For this reason, the recommended dose for methadone should be 10% of the equianalgesic dose of standard opioids.[49] Methadone is not without side effects and drug-to-drug interactions. Respiratory depression and conditions associated with a prolonged QT interval are significant complications of methadone and may cause death. Toxic effects of methadone can be reversed with Naloxone or the longer-acting antagonist Naltrexone.

EQUIANALGESIC DOSES OF OPIOIDS

The appropriate opioid selection requires knowledge about dosage guidelines, the route of administration and potential side effects of various drugs. Critically ill patients frequently become unstable and may not tolerate specific analgesics. Clinicians traditionally use equianalgesic opioid conversion tables to calculate equivalent doses of two different analgesic medications. These tables, however, have limitations and tend to oversimplify opioid-to-opioid conversion, which may lead to ineffective pain management or toxic drug effects.[52] Using evidence based equianalgesic opioid dose ratios considers the bioavailability of the drug which may change from patient to patient (**Table 6**).[53] Most bioavailability research has included patients with chronic pain, further research is needed to guide clinicians in managing analgesia rotation for acutely ill patients.

OPIOID ANTAGONISTS

Drugs that block opioid receptors are referred to as antagonists; they have a high affinity but low efficacy for the receptor. Naloxone and naltrexone are the common opioid antagonists and work on all three opioid receptors, Mu, Kappa and Delta, by preventing their activation by opioids. Both naloxone and naltrexone work centrally and peripherally but in different ways. Naloxone (narcan) given parenterally has a rapid onset of action with a short duration. It is useful to reverse acute opioid effects, mainly respiratory depression, but because of its short half-life, a "re-narcotization" may develop so continued patient assessment and additional doses of naloxone may be required. Naltrexone is administered orally and has a long half-life. It is often used in the long-term treatment of post opioid addition syndromes by relieving symptoms such as anxiety and depression.

NONOPIOIDS AND ADJUVANT ANALGESICS

The inflammatory response often accompanying tissue damage, and hence pain, can be modified by specific medications. Medications that break the inflammatory cycle include nonsteroidal anti-inflammatory drugs (ibuprofen, naprocin), analgesics such as acetaminophen and aspirin or by blocking the enzyme, cyclooxygenase, required for prostaglandin synthesis (ie, COX inhibitors). Anticonvulsants such as gabapentin (Neruontin) and tegretol slow nerve transmission and stabilize "twitchy" nerve membranes, while tricyclic antidepressants interfere with the reuptake of neurotransmitters. Baclofen interferes with transmission of nociceptive impulses and treats pain associated with muscle spasm. Local anesthetics, such as lidocaine and bupivacaine, block nerve transmission along the peripheral nerves.

CLINICAL CHALLENGES OF TREATING PAIN IN OBESE PATIENTS

The obese patient experiences pain from many factors in addition to the traditional incision and procedural pain that often accompany critical illness. In addition to acute pain, the obese patient may also be experiencing chronic pain from arthritis, fibromyalgia, muscle pain, and headaches. The inability of an obese patient to

Table 6 Equianalgesic dose ratios (EDR)	
Commonly Used Opioids for Critically Ill Patients	**EDR**
IV Morphine to PO Morphine	1:2–3
IV Morphine to IV Fentanyl	50–100:1
IV Morphine to IV Hydromorphone	4–7:1
IV Fentanyl to TD Fentanyl	1:1
Hydromorphone to Morphine	7–11:1

Data from Refs.[49,52,53]

self-reposition along with the decrease in blood circulation of adipose tissue puts this population at high risk for developing painful pressure ulcers. Also, folds of skin create a moist environment and may lead to fungal infections and further skin irritation.

Gaining vascular and epidural access in obese patients is often difficult. Central vascular access in obese patients is difficult due to obscure landmarks, the depth of the vessel and the distorted angle of insertion.[46] Skin folds and the inability to adequately position a patient on their side may impede epidural catheter insertion and maintenance.[54] Both indwelling central intravenous and epidural catheters may interfere with activity and increase the risk of infection. Bariatric equipment including beds with a trapeze and low flow air mattresses and transfer devices need to be readily available to prevent the complications of immobility and to prevent injury to the health care team.

SUMMARY

Studies in analgesic pharmacokinetics in obesity remain limited. Appropriate and successful pain management for obese patients entails an understanding of the clinical pharmacology of opioid and nonopioid analgesics and of drug distribution and elimination patterns in obese patients. Drug distribution to lean and fat tissue differs. The loading dose of drugs that are distributed to lean tissues should be base on IBW. For drugs that are distributed primarily to lean but partially to fat tissue, the loading dose should be calculated by using IBW plus a percentage of total body weight. Loading doses for drugs that are equally distributed to lean and fat tissues or mainly fat tissue should be based on ABW. The maintenance dosage depends on the patient's ability to clear the drug.

Pain is a universal phenomenon that does not discriminate by size. Regardless of a patient's weight, an individualized plan of pain management must include selecting the appropriate analgesics, giving the right dose along with developing a dosing schedule to minimize side effects while maximizing pain relief. Nurses play a prominent role in determining the most effective pain management strategy so must understand pharmacokinetics and be alert to the types of pain and how pain affects individuals differently. The obese patient population is not unlike any other group of patients. All require consistent, ongoing assessment and evaluation of interventions to maximize outcomes and improve quality of life.

ACKNOWLEDGMENTS

Special thanks to Trish Seifert, RN, MSN, CNOR, CRNFA, for her invaluable vision, support and guidance.

REFERENCES

1. Ogden CL, Carroll MD, Curtin LR, et al. Prevalence of overweight and obesity in the United States, 1999–2004. JAMA 2006;295(13):1549–55.
2. Buchwald H, Avidor Y, Braunwald E, et al. Bariatric surgery: a systematic review and meta-analysis. JAMA 2004;292(14):1724–37.
3. Rohrer JE, Adamson SC, Barnes D, et al. Obesity and general pain in patients utilizing family medicine: should pain standards call for referral of obese patients to weight management programs? Qual Manag Health Care 2008;17(3):204–9.
4. El-Solh A, Sikka P, Bozkanat E, et al. Morbid obesity in the medical ICU. Chest 2001;120(6):1989–97.

5. Nguyen NT, Root J, Zainabadi K, et al. Accelerated growth of bariatric surgery with the introduction of minimally invasive surgery. Arch Surg 2005;140(12): 1198–202 [discussion: 1203].
6. Lopez PP, Patel NA, Koche LS. Outpatient complications encountered following Roux-en-Y gastric bypass. Med Clin North Am 2007;91(3):471–83, xii.
7. Luber SD, Fischer DR, Venkat A. Care of the bariatric surgery patient in the emergency department. J Emerg Med 2008;34(1):13–20.
8. Wolf AM, Colditz GA. Current estimates of the economic cost of obesity in the United States. Obes Res 1998;6(2):97–106.
9. Akinnusi ME, Pineda LA, El Solh AA. Effect of obesity on intensive care morbidity and mortality: a meta-analysis. Crit Care Med 2008;36(1):151–8.
10. Coley KC, Williams BA, DaPos SV, et al. Retrospective evaluation of unanticipated admissions and readmissions after same day surgery and associated costs. J Clin Anesth 2002;14(5):349–53.
11. Apfelbaum JL, Chen C, Mehta SS, et al. Postoperative pain experience: results from a national survey suggest postoperative pain continues to be undermanaged. Anesth Analg 2003;97(2):534–40, table of contents.
12. American Society of Anesthesiologists Task Force on Acute Pain Management. Practice guidelines for acute pain management in the perioperative setting: an updated report by the American Society of Anesthesiologists Task Force on Acute Pain Management. Anesthesiology 2004;100(6):1573–81.
13. Puntillo K, Weiss SJ. Pain: its mediators and associated morbidity in critically ill cardiovascular surgical patients. Nurs Res 1994;43(1):31–6.
14. Polomano RC, Dunwoody CJ, Krenzischek DA, et al. Perspective on pain management in the 21st century. Pain Manag Nurs 2008;9(Suppl 1):s3–10.
15. Carr DB, Goudas LC. Acute pain. Lancet 1999;353(9169):2051–8.
16. Chen E, Craske MG, Katz ER, et al. Pain-sensitive temperament: does it predict procedural distress and response to psychological treatment among children with cancer? J Pediatr Psychol 2000;25(4):269–78.
17. Kim H, Neubert JK, San Miguel A, et al. Genetic influence on variability in human acute experimental pain sensitivity associated with gender, ethnicity and psychological temperament. Pain 2004;109(3):488–96.
18. Ranger M, Campbell-Yeo M. Temperament and pain response: a review of the literature. Pain Manag Nurs 2008;9(1):2–9.
19. Miller C, Newton SE. Pain perception and expression: the influence of gender, personal self-efficacy, and lifespan socialization. Pain Manag Nurs 2006;7(4): 148–52.
20. Caldwell J, Hart-Johnson T, Green CR. Body mass index and quality of life: examining blacks and whites with chronic pain. J Pain 2009;10(1):60–7.
21. Melzack R. Pain and the neuromatrix in the brain. J Dent Educ 2001;65(12): 1378–82.
22. Melzack R, Wall PD. Pain mechanisms: a new theory. Science 1965;150(699): 971–9.
23. Copstead LE, Banasik JL. Pathophysiology. St. Louis (MO): Elsevier Saunders; 2005.
24. Polomano RC, Rathmell JP, Krenzischek DA, et al. Emerging trends and new approaches to acute pain management. Pain Manag Nurs 2008;9(Suppl 1):s33–41.
25. Helms JE, Barone CP. Physiology and treatment of pain. Crit Care Nurse 2008; 28(6):38–49, quiz 50.
26. Ogunnaike BO, Jones SB, Jones DB, et al. Anesthetic considerations for bariatric surgery. Anesth Analg 2002;95(6):1793–805.

27. Schumann R, Jones SB, Ortiz VE, et al. Best practice recommendations for anesthetic perioperative care and pain management in weight loss surgery. Obes Res 2005;13(2):254–66.
28. Herr K, Coyne PJ, Key T, et al. Pain assessment in the nonverbal patient: position statement with clinical practice recommendations. Pain Manag Nurs 2006;7(2):44–52.
29. Puntillo KA, White C, Morris AB, et al. Patients' perceptions and responses to procedural pain: results from Thunder Project II. Am J Crit Care 2001;10(4): 238–51.
30. Dunwoody CJ, Krenzischek DA, Pasero C, et al. Assessment, physiological monitoring, and consequences of inadequately treated acute pain. Pain Manag Nurs 2008;9(Suppl 1):s11–21.
31. Payen JF, Bru O, Bosson JL, et al. Assessing pain in critically ill sedated patients by using a behavioral pain scale. Crit Care Med 2001;29(12):2258–63.
32. Gelinas C, Fillion L, Puntillo KA, et al. Validation of the critical-care pain observation tool in adult patients. Am J Crit Care 2006;15(4):420–7.
33. McCaffery M, Pasero C. Assessment: underlying complexities, misconceptions, and practical tools. In: McCaffery M, Pasero C, editors. Pain clinical manual. 2nd edition. St. Louis (MO): Mosby; 1999. p. 35–102.
34. Hurst S, Blanco K, Boyle D, et al. Bariatric implications of critical care nursing. Dimens Crit Care Nurs 2004;23(2):76–83.
35. Alexander JK. The cardiomyopathy of obesity. Prog Cardiovasc Dis 1985;27(5): 325–34.
36. Gallagher SM. Obesity and the skin in the critical care setting. Crit Care Nurs Q 2002;25(1):69–75.
37. Benumof JL. Obesity, sleep apnea, the airway and anesthesia. Curr Opin Anaesthesiol 2004;17(1):21–30.
38. Ahmad S, Nagle A, McCarthy RJ, et al. Postoperative hypoxemia in morbidly obese patients with and without obstructive sleep apnea undergoing laparoscopic bariatric surgery. Anesth Analg 2008;107(1):138–43.
39. Bray GA. Pathophysiology of obesity. Am J Clin Nutr 1992;55(Suppl 2):488S–94S.
40. Passannante AN, Rock P. Anesthetic management of patients with obesity and sleep apnea. Anesthesiol Clin North America 2005;23(3):479–91, vii.
41. Charlebois D, Wilmoth D. Critical care of patients with obesity. Crit Care Nurse 2004;24(4):19–27 [quiz: 28–9].
42. Rowland M, Tozer TN. Distribution. In: Roland M, Tozer TN, editors. Clinical pharmacokinetics concepts applications. 3rd edition. Baltimore (MD): Williams & Wilkins; 1995. p. 135–55.
43. Cheymol G. Effects of obesity on pharmacokinetics implications for drug therapy. Clin Pharmacokinet 2000;39(3):215–31.
44. Shibutani K, Inchiosa MA Jr, Sawada K, et al. Pharmacokinetic mass of fentanyl for postoperative analgesia in lean and obese patients. Br J Anaesth 2005;95(3): 377–83.
45. Lee JB, Winstead PS, Cook AM. Pharmacokinetic alterations in obesity. Orthopedics 2006;29(11):984–8.
46. Pieracci FM, Barie PS, Pomp A. Critical care of the bariatric patient. Crit Care Med 2006;34(6):1796–804.
47. Salazar DE, Corcoran GB. Predicting creatinine clearance and renal drug clearance in obese patients from estimated fat-free body mass. Am J Med 1988;84(6): 1053–60.
48. Krenzischek DA, Dunwoody CJ, Polomano RC, et al. Pharmacotherapy for acute pain: implications for practice. Pain Manag Nurs 2008;9(Suppl 1):s22–32.

49. Trescot AM, Datta S, Lee M, et al. Opioid pharmacology. Pain Physician 2008; 11(Suppl 2):s133–53.
50. Shibutani K, Inchiosa MA Jr, Sawada K, et al. Accuracy of pharmacokinetic models for predicting plasma fentanyl concentrations in lean and obese surgical patients: derivation of dosing weight ("pharmacokinetic mass"). Anesthesiology 2004;101(3):603–13.
51. Levi D, Goodman ER, Patel M, et al. Critical care of the obese and bariatric surgical patient. Crit Care Clin 2003;19(1):11–32.
52. Anderson R, Saiers JH, Abram S, et al. Accuracy in equianalgesic dosing: conversion dilemmas. J Pain Symptom Manage 2001;21(5):397–406.
53. Patanwala AE, Duby J, Waters D, et al. Opioid conversions in acute care. Ann Pharmacother 2007;41(2):255–66.
54. Brodsky JB, Lemmens HJ. Regional anesthesia and obesity. Obes Surg 2007; 17(9):1146–9.

Sedation Considerations for the Nonintubated Obese Patient in Critical Care

Mark Welliver, DNP, CRNA, ARNP[a],*, Michele Bednarzyk, MN, FNP, BC[b,c]

KEYWORDS

- Obese • Sedation • Critical care • Obstructive sleep apnea
- Respiratory depression

Obese patients present unique considerations and challenges in critical care units, especially when sedation is required. Obesity is defined as a body mass index greater than 30 kg/m^2.[1] Sedation of the obese patient may be required in emergency departments, ICUs, interventional radiology, surgical suites, and endoscopy units. A primary concern during sedation procedures is patient safety. Maintenance of airway patency and ventilation therefore are of paramount importance. The respiratory status of critically ill obese patients is a primary concern when sedation is administered. Critically ill patients may or may not be intubated and mechanically ventilated. Given the significant confounding conditions that necessitated their admission to critical care units, the sedation of nonintubated obese patients is an imposing challenge. Knowledge of the anatomy, physiology, and pathophysiology associated with obesity, airway management, and sedation agents is essential to prepare one to care for these patients safely and effectively.

GOALS OF SEDATION

Sedation is not a fixed state but rather is a continuum of central nervous system depression induced by pharmacologic agents. Three categories of this continuum have been identified: light, moderate, and deep sedation.[2] The hallmark signs of each depth of sedation are listed in **Table 1**. It is preferable to deliver only light to

[a] School of Nurse Anesthesia, Harris College of Nursing and Health Sciences, Texas Christian University, Fort Worth, TX 76109, USA
[b] Brooks College of Health, School of Nursing, University North Florida, 1 UNF Drive, Jacksonville, FL 32224, USA
[c] Volunteers in Medicine-Jacksonville, Jacksonville, FL, USA
* Corresponding author.
E-mail address: m.welliver@tcu.edu (M. Welliver).

Crit Care Nurs Clin N Am 21 (2009) 341–352
doi:10.1016/j.ccell.2009.07.001
0899-5885/09/$ – see front matter © 2009 Published by Elsevier Inc.

moderate sedation and to avoid deep sedation. The goals of light and moderate sedation include maintaining a patent airway, protective reflexes, and response to verbal
stimuli. Despite the hallmark signs associated with light and moderate sedation,
studies have found deep levels of sedation frequently occur during sedative procedures.[3] At any level of sedation, airway compromise is more likely to occur in obese
patients because of anatomic and physiologic alterations.

AIRWAY ANATOMY

The airway in the nonobese patient is maintained in the supine position. In the normal
airway, the oral pharyngeal muscles, even with relaxation, maintain airway patency
and allow air flow (**Fig. 1**). In contrast, the obese patient's airway has redundant tissue
that contributes to narrowing of the oral pharynx which worsens in the supine position
(**Fig. 2**). Obesity is a significant risk factor for oxygen desaturation, and any suppression of respiratory function mandates judicious sedation titration and vigilant monitoring.[4] A recent study found similar frequent oxygen desaturations in obese
patients with and without obstructive sleep apnea (OSA).[5] OSA heightens concern
when sedating obese patients because it foretells of airway compromise. Its presence,
causative mechanisms, and the degree and the use of continuous positive airway
pressure (CPAP) need to be known. Often a patient's spouse will disclose a history
of snoring and breathing pauses even in the absence of a formal diagnosis of OSA.
If a patient experiences airway occlusion during normal sleep, it should be expected
with sedation.

OBSTRUCTIVE SLEEP APNEA

OSA is more common in obese patients than in patients of ideal weight. OSA is diagnosed with documented periods of 10 seconds or more of total cessation of airflow
despite respiratory efforts.[6] Overnight sleep studies using polysomnography formally
confirm the diagnosis. Such individuals usually have floppy upper airways and fat
deposition in the lateral pharyngeal walls.[7] The inherent narrowing of the obese airway
is worsened by the relaxation of the pharyngeal musculature and posterior displacement of the tongue that occurs naturally during sleep, especially in the supine position.
These factors coupled with the dynamics of ventilatory flow converge to occlude the
airway. A flow dynamic called the "Bernoulli effect" is the increased gas flow velocity
and associated lower pressure at an area of constriction in a tube (**Fig. 3**). The lower
pressure at the site of a narrowing results in partial or complete collapse and obstruction of the airway. CPAP masks raise the airway pressure to counteract the Bernoulli
effect. Stalford[8] also described a Starling resistor model that reflects higher
surrounding tissue pressures that contribute to the airway collapse. Review of the literature reveals multiple sites of obstruction.[9] It is likely that multiple sites and factors, in
addition to the physics of flow, are responsible for OSA. Upper airway

Table 1		
Hallmark signs of sedation		
Sedation Level	**Hallmark Signs**	
Light	Ptosis, slurred speech	
Moderate	Arousable to loud voice	
Deep	Responsive to deep pain only. May have airway occlusion or apnea. May need airway assistance or support.	

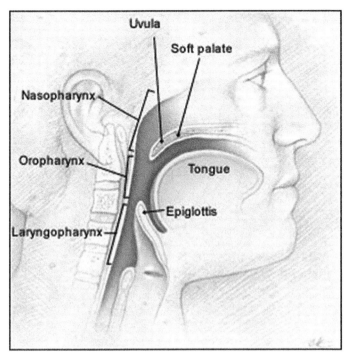

Fig. 1. Normal airway. (© Christy Krames, 2002. *Reprinted* with permission.)

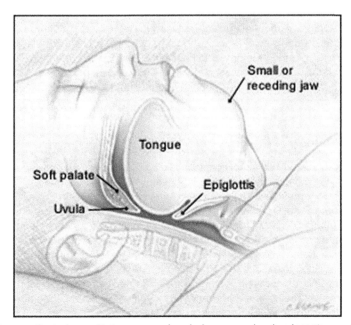

Fig. 2. Obese patient airway. Note narrowed oral pharynx and redundant tissues. (© Christy Krames, 2002. *Reprinted* with permission.)

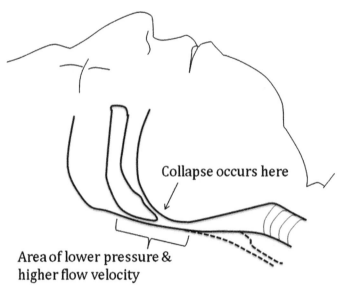

Collapse occurs here

Area of lower pressure &
higher flow velocity

Fig. 3. Bernoulli effect. Note decreased pressure at constriction which tends to collapse airway. (*Modified from* **Fig. 2**, Obese patient airway. © Christy Krames, 2002. *Reprinted with permission.*)

mechanoreceptors that dilate the airway in response to lower airway pressures may be less responsive in the patient who has OSA.[10]

The airway occlusion that occurs in OSA causes intermittent breathing cessation. These apneic episodes raise arterial CO_2 and lower arterial O_2 levels. This change disrupts normal sleep patterns by partially awakening the patient, and a deep breath is initiated. Rapid eye movement pattern sleep is decreased, leading to fatigue and limited alertness during awake hours. Patients who have OSA are sleep deprived, often falling asleep during the day, and have difficulty focusing attention. Sleep deprivation and fatigue make patients who have OSA more susceptible to sedative agents. Even without the diagnosis of OSA, obese patients are at risk for airway compromise during sedation.[5,11]

ALTERED PHYSIOLOGY

Obesity is associated with significant physiologic changes. Awake, spontaneously breathing obese patients have decreased chest wall compliance and often have inefficient respiratory muscles. The work of breathing increases with increasing obesity and is associated with increased O_2 consumption and CO_2 production.[12] Greater diaphragmatic effort is required for effective ventilation in obese patients than in patients of lesser weight. A large abdominal compartment that pushes upward, especially in the supine position, makes ventilation and diaphragmatic excursion more difficult. The supine position displaces the abdominal contents and compresses the thoracic compartment. With increasing weight, intra-abdominal pressure is increased, and inspiratory reserve volume, expiratory reserve volume, functional residual capacity, vital capacity, and total lung capacity are all decreased when compared with normal-weight patients.[13] These changes usually are attributed to mass loading of the chest wall and splinting of the diaphragm by thoracic and abdominal adipose tissue. Airway closure occurs during normal tidal ventilation, producing air-trapping, shunting, and a lower P_{AO_2} than would be expected in a similar patient of normal weight. In morbidly obese patients (BMI >40), cardiac output, systemic and pulmonary artery pressure, and left and right ventricular pressure are all increased. These changes manifest as arterial hypertension, ischemic heart disease, right and left heart failure, and cardiomegaly.[14]

Positioning

Obesity is associated with high intra-abdominal pressure and decreased lung volumes. These decreases are worse in the presence of sedation and anesthesia. If the abdomen is compressed, the diaphragm is displaced, and chest wall movement is restricted. Relieving the high intra-abdominal pressure increases functional residual capacity and improves oxygenation. This relief of pressure can be accomplished either by lifting the panniculus or by raising the patient's back. Extremely obese patients should not be permitted to lie completely flat or in Trendelenburg position during sedation. At a minimum, they should be placed in the semi-Fowler's position. One must ensure, however, that improved oxygenation is not offset by decreased cardiac output because of decreased venous return. Lithotomy position also displaces the abdominal contents against the diaphragm, reducing lung volumes. Lithotomy and Trendelenburg positions accentuate all the negative physiologic effects of the supine position and should be avoided if possible. If lithotomy or Trendelenburg position is required, controlled ventilation with an endotracheal tube should be used. A semi-recumbent position should be maintained during postsedation convalescence.[5]

Monitoring

Light and moderate levels of sedation require the maintenance of arousability and airway patency. Continuous, thorough assessment of respiratory rate, rhythm, depth, and protective reflexes (cough, swallowing) must be conducted. Ease of ventilation, free of snoring or grunting, needs to be maintained. Nurses monitoring the patient should not be required to participate in other activities that will distract them from these monitoring tasks. Pulse oximetry, ECG, pulse, and blood pressure also should be monitored continually and documented frequently (usually every 5 minutes or as dictated by institutional policy).[4]

Airway Management

Challenges with the obese patient include an airway that is prone to collapse and occlusion. Obese patients often snore and have OSA, forewarning of the greater likelihood of airway compromise during sedation procedures. Suppression of ventilation, apnea, and laryngospasm may occur during sedation procedures. Sedation causes decreased respiratory drive, rate, and depth. The administration of supplemental oxygen raises the inspired oxygen fraction entering the lungs even during shallow breaths. The higher inspired oxygen may give a false sense of security by maintaining a high pulse oximetry value despite significant hypoxemia. Hypoxemia is defined as an arterial oxygen tension (P_{AO_2}) lower than expected for a given inspired oxygen concentration (F_{IO_2}). A pulse oximeter will display an oxygen saturation of 100% if the P_{AO_2} is 100 mm Hg to 250 mm Hg or higher. Normal lung function inspiring 50% oxygen would be expected to produce a P_{AO_2} of 250 mm Hg. A P_{AO_2} of 100 mm Hg while breathing 50% oxygen represents significant pulmonary dysfunction, but a pulse oximeter is not capable of identifying this ventilation/perfusion mismatch. Elevated P_{AO_2} levels also occur with hypoventilation. P_{CO_2} levels are not routinely, or accurately, measured during sedative procedures. Severely elevated P_{CO_2} levels produce somnolence and worsening hypoventilation and contributes to respiratory failure.[15]

Laryngospasm is a natural reflex that closes the glottic opening of the airway to prevent aspiration. It usually is followed by a forceful cough that stretches and relaxes the vocal cords to allow the expelling of the offending stimulus (eg, oral secretions). Sedation can decrease the patient's ability to swallow and cough, allowing secretions to stimulate laryngospasm. A rocking movement of the patient's chest without ventilatory exchange should alert one to the incidence of obstruction and possible laryngospasm. A chin lift and jaw thrust sometimes is enough to restore airway patency and ventilation. If these maneuvers are ineffective, a chin lift while tightly holding a bag/mask unit on the patient's face with positive-pressure ventilation may end the laryngospasm. Two hands on the mask and jaw may be needed while another person lightly administers positive pressure (<20 cm H_2O) ventilation by squeezing the bag of the bag-mask-valve resuscitator. A last alternative to end resistant laryngospasm is the administration of 10 to 20 mg of succinylcholine, a short-acting muscle relaxant. The patient will require effective artificial ventilation until the succinylcholine effects are gone and the sedation is reversed or wears off.[16]

PREPARATION

Delineation of tasks and a plan of care need to be established before sedation. Preparation for sedation includes gathering all necessary equipment ahead of time. An oxygen supply, preferably with a back-up source, along with administration devices such as nasal cannulae, a face mask, oral airways, nasal trumpets, and bag-mask-valve resuscitator need to be prepared. If the patient uses a CPAP mask at home, it should be used during sedation procedures. Because of the unique difficulties associated with sedating obese patients, consideration should be given to positioning, monitoring, airway management, drug selection and dose, and plan for loss of airway and ventilation.[4]

DRUG TITRATION

It is desirable to have intravenous (IV) fluid flowing slowly to carry the administered drugs and maintain IV patency. Needle piercing of heparin lock IV access followed by flushes is cumbersome, inefficient, and may interfere with any procedure being conducted that requires sedation. Universal precautions should be maintained during all sedation procedures, including drug administration. When sedation is administered, it is important to remain cognizant of the dose, onset time, and peak onset time of each agent. The expected drug effects often are enhanced in obese patients because of their anatomy, physiology, and concomitant illness. The anatomic and physiologic considerations previously described, along with alterations in drug binding, distribution, and clearance, encourage slow, judicious administration of sedatives. Obese patients have a greater volume of distribution for lipophilic drugs and thus these drugs have a longer duration. Protein binding of sedation drugs is altered and may increase or decrease plasma concentrations.[17] Administered doses should be decreased from recommended per kilogram dosages to prevent overdose. Obese patients often have normal lean body mass with excessive adipose tissue. Dosing drugs to total body weight results in large amounts of administered drug and likely excessive effects. Small doses should be administered, and time should be allowed for peak effect to occur. Assessment of drug effect and re-administration as needed offer the best regimen for sedation. Administering sedative drugs too frequently may contribute to "stacking" of the drug, with the inevitable peak effect higher than desired. Additionally, the concomitant administration of narcotic drugs with sedative agents causes a synergistic effect.[18] (Synergism occurs when the total effect of the drugs exceeds that which would be expected if the effects of the individual drugs were added.) The following sections present a brief overview of commonly used sedative drugs.

Sedation Drugs

Midazolam (Versed) is a benzodiazepine drug with effects similar to those of diazepam (Valium) but with a shorter duration and faster clearance from the body. For this reason, midazolam often is the drug of choice for sedation procedures. Midazolam has respiratory depressant effects and can cause loss of airway patency and ventilation. Its effects are prolonged in the obese.[11,17]

Propofol (Diprivan) is a sedative agent at lower doses and is a general anesthetic at higher doses. Because of its quick onset and quick offset, it frequently is used for sedative procedures. Propofol has potent respiratory depressant effects and must be administered judiciously. Small incremental doses of propofol may transition the patient from light or moderate sedation to deep sedation or general anesthesia. Propofol possess a narrow therapeutic window, and small dose increments may easily cause overdose (**Fig. 4**). Other considerations for the use of propofol include its preparation as a lipid emulsion that supports bacterial growth. The presence of preservatives slows but does not prevent bacterial growth after contamination. Contamination may occur merely by drawing the drug from its vial, and this action has been identified as a frequent cause of hospital-acquired sepsis.[19] Hyperlipidemia from continuous infusions for more than 24 hours has been documented and may aggravate existing hyperlipidemia in obese patients.[20] Propofol syndrome is another unique consideration associated with propofol. Propofol syndrome is characterized by metabolic acidosis, rhabdomyolysis, renal failure, and cardiac failure, primarily in critically ill and children.[21] Hyperlipidemia and propofol syndrome are more likely with extended use than with propofol sedation of short duration.

Fospropofol (Lusedra) is a newly approved aqueous prodrug of propofol. A prodrug is a nonactive drug that is similar to an active drug but requires a metabolic or

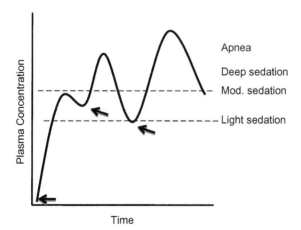

Fig. 4. Level of sedation varies with drug dosage and time. The therapeutic index is between the dotted lines. *Arrows* show propofol bolus administration followed by effect.

enzymatic alteration in the body before it can exert an effect. Fospropofol must be converted by enzymes in the body to the active propofol molecules before sedative effects occur. This enzymatic conversion occurs slowly over 5 to 10 minutes and lasts approximately 20 to 30 minutes after a bolus injection. Plasma levels of propofol converted from fospropofol reach a more steady therapeutic level than boluses of regular propofol (Diprivan) **(Fig. 5)**. The effects of fospropofol therefore are less dramatic than those of propofol, because plasma levels are released slowly. Bolus doses of 6.5 mg/kg have been found to offer effective moderate sedation with few incidences of airway compromise. As a new drug that slowly converts to propofol, fospropofol may offer benefit for sedation procedures in obese patients. One should not be tempted to give additional doses of fospropofol because of its delayed onset and lesser effects compared with propofol (Diprivan). Additional doses of fospropofol risk stacking of the drug, resulting in an overdose because of the delayed enzymatic conversion process.[22]

Dexmedetomidine (Precedex) is an alpha$_2$ receptor agonist that works in the brain to produce sedative, analgesic, and sympatholytic effects. It is administered by intravenous infusion and not by bolus. The onset of sedation occurs within 5 minutes and does not alter respiratory rate or rhythm. Undesirable effects of dexmedetomidine—hypotension and bradycardia—are related to the alpha$_2$ receptor agonism.[23]

Etomidate is a drug in its own unique class. It is a sedative/hypnotic drug at low doses and an anesthetic induction agent at higher doses. Etomidate possess desirable properties including hemodynamic and respiratory stability. Low doses of etomidate cause little or no suppression of respiratory rate and rhythm. Although it has been used successfully as a sedative agent, adrenal suppression caused by this drug may limit its application in critically ill patients.[24]

Adjunct Drugs

Narcotics are analgesic adjuncts sometimes administered with sedative drugs. Narcotics and sedative drugs display synergism when administered together: the combined respiratory depressant effects of each are increased when administered concomitantly. Narcotics lessen the response of the central nervous system respiratory drive related to increased CO_2 levels in the blood and lower the respiratory rate

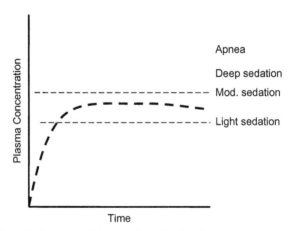

Fig. 5. Effect of single fospropofol bolus. Note steady plasma concentration within therapeutic index over time.

Table 2
Intravenous drugs frequently administered for sedation procedures

Drug	Class	Approximate Dose (70 kg Ideal Body Weight)	Onset	Duration	Primary Metabolism
Midazolam	Tranquilizer	1–4 mg	1–3 min	1–2 hours	Hepatic
Lorazepam	Tranquilizer	0.5–2mg	1–3 min	4+ hours	Hepatic
Diazepam	Tranquilizer	1–4 mg	1–3 min	6+ hours	Hepatic
Demeral	Opioid	25–100 mg	1–3 min	2–4 hours	Hepatic
Morphine	Opioid	5–10 mg	1–3 min	4 hours	Hepatic
Fentanyl	Opioid	50–100 μg	1–3 min	1–1.5 hour	Hepatic
Propofol	Sedative/hypnotic	5–10 mg Infuse at 10–25 μg/kg/min	1–3 min	5–10 min	Hepatic
Etomidate	Sedative/hypnotic	1–2 mg	1–3 min	5–10 min	Hepatic, plasma enzymes
Dexmedetomidine	Sedative/hypnotic	1 μg/kg over 10 minutes. Infuse at 1–7 μg/kg/min	5–10 min	Ultrashort upon drip cessation	Hepatic
Ketamine	Dissociative	10–20 mg	1–3 min	10–20 min	Hepatic
Fospropofol	Sedative/hypnotic	6.5 mg/kg	5–10 min	20–30 min	Hepatic

and depth. Narcotics also relax pharyngeal musculature, predisposing obese patients to further airway collapse. The increased adipose tissue and co-existing morbidities contribute to altered durations of these drugs and the exaggerated respiratory depressant effects.[17]

Although narcotics do not directly lower blood pressure, they tend to lower heart rate and attenuate sympathetic nervous system tone. Critically ill patients may have elevated blood pressure because of catecholamines secreted in response to stress, anxiety, and pain. Narcotics, by lessening the stimuli responsible for catecholamine release, may lower blood pressure indirectly. The heart rate–lowering effect along with decreased blood pressure must be considered when using narcotics in critically ill patients. The narcotics most often used are meperidine, morphine, and, occasionally, fentanyl (**Table 2**).

Ketamine is a dissociative anesthetic that does not depress respirations. Ketamine acts on N-methyl-D-aspartate receptors in the central nervous system, altering normal consciousness. Ketamine is rarely given alone because it may cause hallucinations and agitation (**Table 3**). Midazolam usually is given along with ketamine to produce a catatonic state that is well tolerated. At higher doses ketamine may increase airway secretions and heart rate.[25]

Reversal Drugs

Both benzodiazepines and narcotics may be reversed with antagonist drugs. Midazolam is reversible with flumazenil (Romazicon) (0.2 mg IV every 1–2 minutes to a maximum of 3 mg/hr). Flumazenil will bind to the γ-aminobutyric acid (GABA) receptor in the central nervous system. Flumazenil attaches to GABA receptors and prevents midazolam from attaching to those receptors and producing its sedative effects. Sedation is reversed by flumazenil within 1 to 2 minutes. Flumazenil may precipitate seizure activity in patients who chronically take GABA agonists such as diazepam (Valium) or zolpidem (Ambien, Zoldem). Narcotics are reversible with naloxone (Narcan) (0.04–2 mg every 1–2 minutes). Return of spontaneous respirations of adequate rate, rhythm, and depth along with appropriate oxygenation and CO_2 clearance indicates effective reversal of narcotics. It is important to note that naloxone

Table 3 Comparison of sedative drug clinical effects			
Drug	Respiratory Depression	Hemodynamic Depression	Central Nervous System Depression
Midazolam	+	+	+++
Diazepine	+	+	+++
Lorazepam	+	+	+++
Meperidine	++	+	+
Morphine	++	+	+
Propofol	+++	+++	++++
Etomidate	−	−	++++
Dexmedetomidine	−	+	+++
Ketamine	−	−	−[a]
Fospropofol	+	+	++

Key: − None to minimal; + mild; ++ moderate; +++ pronounced; ++++ maximal.
[a] May cause agitation.

effects wear off in approximately 20 minutes and longer acting narcotic effects may return to suppress respirations. Patients who receive sedative or narcotic reversal drugs need continued close monitoring and assessment.

SUMMARY

Sedation of the obese patient is complicated by altered anatomy and physiology predisposing these often critically ill patients to respiratory suppression, airway obstruction, hypoxemia, and hypercarbia. The critical illness that necessitated their admission to the critical care unit increases the risks associated with sedation of the non-intubated obese patient. Sedation procedures should not be rushed and always conducted in a well-organized setting with appropriate airway support including suction, suction catheters, oxygen, oxygen delivery devices, and a bag-mask-valve resuscitator. Preparation for immediate airway support, including intubation, should be made before sedation. The obese patient always is a challenge for nursing staff. A thorough understanding of the pathophysiology of obesity, with special consideration for the increased risk of airway occlusion and effects of positioning on respiratory mechanics will allow the safer administration of sedation in this high-risk population.

REFERENCES

1. Spiegel AM, Alving BM. Executive summary of the strategic plan for National Institutes of Health obesity research. Am J Clin Nutr 2005;82:211S–4S.
2. Kost M. Locations and specific conscious sedation procedures. In: Connor M, editor. Manual of conscious sedation. Philadelphia: W.B. Saunders; 1997. p. 176–82.
3. Patel S, Vargo JJ, Khandwala F, et al. Deep sedation occurs frequently during elective endoscopy with meperidine and midazolam. Am J Gastroenterol 2005; 100:2689–95.
4. Somerson SJ, Husted CW, Sicilia MR. Insights into: conscious sedation. Am J Nurs 1995;95(6):26–33.
5. Jain SS, Dhand R. Perioperative treatment of patients with obstructive sleep apnea. Curr Opin Pulm Med 2004;10(6):482–8.
6. Okwuone CO, Po W, Swick JT, et al. Obstructive sleep apnea—implications for procedural sedation. J Radiol Nurs 2006;25:2–6.
7. Hora F, Nápolis LM, Daltro C, et al. Clinical, anthropometric and upper airway anatomic characteristics of obese patients with obstructive sleep apnea syndrome. Respiration 2007;74:517–24.
8. Stalford C. Update for nurse anesthetists. The Starling resistor: a model for explaining and treating obstructive sleep apnea. AANA J 2004;72(2):133–8.
9. Rama AN, Tekwani SH, Kushida CA. Sites of obstruction in obstructive sleep apnea. Chest 2002;122:1139–47.
10. Moos DD. Obstructive sleep apnea and sedation in the endoscopy suite. Gastroenterol Nurs 2007;29(6):456–65.
11. Patil SP, Schneider H, Marxx JJ, et al. Neuromechanical control of upper airway patency during sleep. J Appl Physiol 2007;102(2):547–56.
12. Kress JP, Pohlman AS, Alverdy J, et al. The impact of morbid obesity on oxygen cost of breathing (Vo_{2RESP}) at rest. Am J Respir Crit Care Med 1999;160:883–6.
13. Pelosi P, Croci M, Ravagnan I, et al. Respiratory system mechanics in sedated, paralyzed, morbidly obese patients. J Appl Physiol 1997;82:811–8.
14. Alpert MA. Obesity cardiomyopathy: Pathophysiology and evolution of the clinical syndrome. Am J Med Sci 2001;321(4):225–36.

15. Brodsky JB, Oldroyd M, Winfield HN, et al. Morbid obesity and the prone position: a case report. J Clin Anesth 2001;13:138–40.
16. Ebert TJ, Shankar H, Haake RM. Perioperative considerations for patients with morbid obesity. Anesthesiol Clin 2006;24:621–36.
17. Casati A, Putzu M. Anesthesia in the obese patient: pharmacokinetic considerations. J Clin Anesth 2005;17(2):134–45.
18. Shafer A. Complications of sedation with midazolam in the intensive care unit and a comparison with other sedative regimens. Crit Care Med 1998;26(5):947–56.
19. Bennett SN, McNeil MM, Bland LA, et al. Postoperative infections traced to contamination of an intravenous anesthetic, propofol. N Engl J Med 1995;333: 147–54.
20. Bairaktari A, Raitsiou B, Kokolaki M, et al. Respiratory failure after pneumonectomy in a patient with unknown hyperlipemia. Anesth Analg 2001;93:292–3.
21. Vasile B, Rasulo F, Candiani A, et al. The pathophysiology of propofol infusion syndrome: a simple name for a complex syndrome. Intensive Care Med 2003; 29:1417–25.
22. Welliver M, Rugari S. New drug fospropofol disodium a propofol prodrug. AANA J 2009;77(4):301–8.
23. Precedex. Available at: http://precedex.hospira.com/default.aspx. Accessed March 22, 2009.
24. Keim SM, Erstad BL, Sakles JC, et al. Etomidate for procedural sedation in the emergency room department. Pharmacotherapy 2002;22(5):586–92.
25. Ivani G, Verecillino C, Tonetti F. Ketamine: a new look at an old drug. Minerva Anesthesiol 2003;69:468–71.

Providing Nutrition to Critically Ill Obese Adults: Use of the Nursing Process

Susan Smith, MS, RN, CNS[a],*, Kathleen Fedyszen, RN, BSN[b]

KEYWORDS
• Nursing • Critical care nursing • Critical illness • Nutrition
• Obesity • Enteral nutrition • Nursing process

More than 60 million people or 32 percent of the adult American population are now obese.[1] When obese individuals become ill, they often carry additional burdens of pre-morbid conditions that are associated with increased weight.[2] These conditions can challenge the ability of nurses and other health care providers to ensure adequate nutrition of the obese patient in the face of critical illness.

Malnutrition is a well-known phenomenon in hospitalized patients and is surprisingly common with rates described from 32 to 59 percent in the United States.[3] It may be present on admission or it can develop during the course of an illness; the resultant consequences are well described in the literature.[4]

Nurses use the nursing process when providing care to patients to reach the best possible outcomes for their identified problems and needs. This process can be used when providing nutrition to obese adult critically ill patients through assessment, diagnosis planning, implementation and evaluation. This article follows the nursing process in exploring the unique care processes involved in providing nutrition to critically ill obese adults.

The gastrointestinal tract plays a significant role in humans as a result of being the largest organ of immune function. Delaying and withholding nutrition interrupts this needed function and places patients at great risk for complications associated with malnutrition, such as infection, increased length of stay, hospitalization costs, and mortality.[5] In their database examination of 263,961 inpatient days over two decades, Zizza and colleagues[6] found that obese patients had a longer length of stay than

[a] Critical Care Unit, Texas Health Presbyterian Hospital Plano, 6200 West Parker Road, Plano, TX 75093-7914, USA
[b] Department of Education, Texas Health Presbyterian Hospital Plano, 6200 West Parker Road, Plano, TX 75093-7914, USA
* Corresponding author.
E-mail address: susanqsmith@texashealth.org (S. Smith).

Crit Care Nurs Clin N Am 21 (2009) 353–367
doi:10.1016/j.ccell.2009.07.013
0899-5885/09/$ – see front matter © 2009 Elsevier Inc. All rights reserved.

normal weight patients. This finding has great importance in this day of reduced reimbursement to hospitals.

Obese, critically ill patients are at greater risk for aspiration pneumonia and for difficulty in weaning from mechanical ventilation, resulting from both increased abdominal weight and changes in respiratory mechanics.[2,7] Malnourished patients have muscle mass losses that can impair their mobility and affect the strength of the diaphragm resulting in increased work of breathing.[4] Akinnusi and colleagues[8] reviewed 14 studies involving a total of 62,045 patients and found that the obese patients were not more likely to die but did experience longer periods of mechanical ventilation and intensive care unit (ICU) length of stay.

Delays in feeding can easily occur in the critical care setting. Priorities must be given to alterations that are immediately seen and the effects of malnutrition are not as quickly apparent in the critical care setting.[9] The obese patient is at greater risk than the normal weight patient, when under stress, to develop nutritional depletion particularly for protein-energy malnutrition. This result is because obese individuals often lack adequate protein resources and, when faced with starvation, they will mobilize endogenous lipids as the primary source of fuel.[10]

Providing effective nutrition therapy to critically ill patients involves several processes, including nutrition screening, nutrition assessment, nutrition support and nutrition monitoring. Often unintentional weight loss and Body Mass Index (BMI) are initial screening indicators of the patient's pre-admission nutritional state and they can also be evaluated throughout the patient's admission for ongoing nutritional state.[4]

BMI is an index of weight-for-height that is commonly used to classify weight in adults and is defined as the weight in kilograms divided by the square of the height in meters (kg/m^2). It is not gender specific or age dependent.[11] The World Health Organization has defined weight limits for classification of adults for underweight, normal, overweight and obese as described in **Table 1**.

There are many screening tools available to clinicians to evaluate how at risk a patient is for malnourishment; these tools measure even more variables, although tools specific to critically ill patients and critically ill obese patients have yet to be developed and validated.[4,12] All hospitalized patients should be screened for nutrition within the first 24 hours of admission to meet The Joint Commission (TJC) requirements, which were developed as a way to prevent malnutrition.[3]

Enteral nutrition should be started within the first 24 to 48 hours after admission to the ICU after the patient is adequately fluid resuscitated and hemodynamically stable.[13–15]

Table 1	
WHO International classification of overweight and obesity	
Classification	BMI (kg/m^2)
Underweight	<18.5
Normal weight	18.5–24.99
Overweight	≥25.00
Pre-obese	25.00–29.99
Obese	≥30.00
Obese Class I	30.00–34.99
Obese Class II	35.00–39.99
Obese Class III	≥40.00

Data from WHO 2004.

Patients who require escalating or high dose catecholamines or are hypotensive (mean arterial pressure <60 mmHg) may be prone to developing ischemic bowel, which is a rare (<1%) complication of enteral nutrition so should not be fed until they are stable.[13]

All patients, including those who are obese, who experience delays in receiving nutrition—especially for more than seven days—are at risk for the potentially fatal complication of refeeding syndrome. This problem is manifested by acute fluid and electrolyte disturbances after sustained malnutrition and starvation. Refeeding syndrome occurs when carbohydrates are reintroduced after a period of significant malnutrition or starvation.[16,17] Patients who have a history of alcohol abuse, anorexia, and significant weight loss are at greatest risk.[17]

The most frequent cause of problems in refeeding syndrome is a result of severe hypophosphotemia. When glucose metabolism is re-established, the use of phosphate to manufacture adenosine triphosphate (ATP) is significantly increased to the point that the patient develops a serious serum reduction with resultant complications, such as respiratory distress, heart failure, confusion, seizures and even death. Other causes of refeeding syndrome are hypokalemia, hypomagnesemia, hyperglycemia, and thiamine deficiency.[16]

Patients are also at risk for overfeeding. Obese patients are more likely to have co-morbidities of diabetes and insulin resistance. Overfeeding interferes with control of hyperglycemia. Overfeeding of calories also promotes lipogenesis, placing the patient at risk for development of fatty liver and overall liver dysfunction.[2]

In contrast, providing adequate nutrition can reduce the rate of nosocomial infection, improve wound healing, and decrease mortality.[9] The challenge to the critical care nurse and other practitioners is to provide nutrition in a way that takes into account their unique needs and requirements.

ASSESSMENT

During assessment, the nurse systematically collects data to determine the patient's health status and to identify actual or potential health problems. The assessment should include a careful review of the patient's history and a physical examination. This step includes the analysis of all data and assists with the formulation of a meaningful nursing diagnosis.[18]

There are many parameters to assess and measure the nutritional state of patients. However, some are not appropriate for use in the critical care environment. Typically, the most used measures of an individual's current nutritional state include: BMI, anthropometric parameters, albumin, prealbumin levels, transferrin, total lymphocyte count, and 24-hour urine creatinine clearance.[4,9] None of these have been validated for use in the critical care population.[13] Pre-albumin appears to be the most sensitive indicator of changes in a patient's nutrition state with a half-life of 3 days.[4]

Presence of flatus, stool, or bowel sounds have traditionally been used as hallmarks for readiness to feed and evidence of bowel motility. Even patients with evidence of mild to moderate clinical ileus can be fed enterally, because feeding can improve gut motility and assist in resolution of ileus, while maintaining NPO status can propagate ileus.[13] Tolerance to enteral nutrition can be monitored by patient complaints of pain, discomfort and/or distention, physical examination, passage of flatus and stool, and abdominal radiographs.[13]

Patients who do not require either enteral or parenteral nutrition interventions have an adequate oral intake and they are thought to be able to receive oral intake in the next 24 hours or are under palliative care.[19] Unless the patient's gastrointestinal tract is not functioning, nutrition should be provided through the enteral route.[5] When nutrition is provided in this manner, the nutrients are metabolized and used more physiologically than when provided via the parenteral route.

Parenteral nutrition should be reserved for those who have specific contraindications for enteral nutrition, such as acute pancreatitis, enteric anastamosis, ischemic bowel, enteric fistula, imminent bowel resection, imminent endoscopy, bowel obstruction, high nasogastric (NG) losses, or severe exacerbation of inflammatory bowel disease.[19] Patients who require parenteral nutrition should be reassessed at regular intervals for appropriateness of changing to enteral nutrition.[13]

Use of the enteral route helps to preserve the structure and barrier functions of the gastrointestinal route and its immune function. Enteral nutrition is associated with reduction in sepsis and infectious complications, decrease in ICU length of stay, and its costs are significantly less than parenteral nutrition.[20]

To assess the patient's nutritional needs the most definitive measurements are through measurement of the respiratory quotient (RQ) by indirect calorimetry (IC).[9] However, RQ measurements require the use of specialized equipment that may not be available to all practitioners and hence predictive equations are used.

IC continues to be the gold standard for measuring energy requirements and predicting nutritional needs in the critically ill.[12,15,21] IC measures oxygen consumption (VO_2) and carbon dioxide elimination (VCO_2). There are two methods for measuring VO_2 and VCO_2. The most commonly used method measures pulmonary gas exchange by the patient breathing into a mask, mouthpiece or via the endotracheal tube connected to the IC device for analysis. Another method measures arterial-venous oxygen content and cardiac output with a pulmonary artery catheter. This method applies thermodilution with quantification of hemodynamic parameters using Fick's formula.

Energy expenditure should be measured under resting conditions in critically ill patients. VCO_2 and VO_2 are vital measurements when calculating resting energy expenditure (REE) with the modified Weir equation. Urinary nitrogen is omitted in this shortened formula as this only accounts for less than four percent energy expenditure and has an error rate of one to two percent.[22] Calculation of the REE determines the patient's total daily caloric requirements while at rest.

$$REE \ (kcal/d) \ = \ [(VO_2 \times 3.941) + (VCO_2 \times 1.11) \ \times \ 1440]$$

The RQ, a ratio of carbon dioxide produced to oxygen consumed (VCO_2/VO_2), is a reflection of which nutrients the body is using as fuel.[23] Normal RQ range is 0.7–1.0. RQ values less than 1.0 may be a sign of overfeeding, lipogenesis, and excess CO_2; RQ values greater than 0.7 may suggest technical problems or metabolic causes described below. Care is warranted when interpreting RQ values in the critically ill because stress response, pulmonary disease, acid-base balance, and medications can alter values making them inaccurate.[24]

Although IC is usually considered to be more accurate than using predictive equations, IC is not foolproof and does have limitations. It is essential patients are monitored for the following factors to ensure IC values are accurate. Improperly maintained and calibrated equipment, as well as the presence of system air leaks, such as an endotracheal tube cuff leak, chest tube leak, and bronchopleural fistula, may limit the accuracy of IC.[22]

Factors impacting gas exchange may contribute to erroneous IC values. Main factors include: fluctuating fraction of inspired oxygen (FiO_2) and > 60% FiO_2, dialysis, postoperative anesthesia, high pain level, sedative and analgesic medications, and nutritional support. Other limitations of IC use include having trained staff available to operate equipment and interpret values, the cost of purchasing and maintaining equipment, and poor insurance reimbursement for studies done.[24]

If IC is not available, a predictive equation is used. More than 200 predictive equations have been published, but many are based on healthy, normal weight individuals and frequently overestimate or underestimate the energy requirements of the critically ill.[13] The American Dietetic Association (ADA)[15] recommends use of the 2003 Penn State, Swinamer, and 1992 Ireton-Jones equations in the non-obese critically ill. For critically ill obese patients requiring mechanical ventilation, the ADA[15] recommends use of the 1992 Ireton-Jones or 1998 Penn State predictive equations.

Interestingly, the Canadian Clinical Practice Guidelines (2009) report insufficient data to recommend the use of IC over predictive equations in determining energy requirements for the critically ill. The SCCM/ASPEN Guidelines from 2009 suggest using caution when using predictive equations since they are less accurate in estimating energy requirements (**Box 1**).

The ADA (2006) strongly discourages the use of the Harris-Benedict, with or without activity and stress factors, the 1997 Ireton-Jones, and the Fick predictive equations in the critically ill population because of inaccuracy. Studies indicate the Harris-Benedict equation has a 17%–67% range of accuracy and commonly overestimates and underestimates energy requirements in the critically ill.[24]

Literature shows the 1997 Ireton-Jones equation overestimated energy needs in 52% of mechanically ventilated patients, while having a tendency to underestimate the needs of other patients.[24] Additionally, the ADA (2006) does not support the use of the Mifflin-St. Jeor predictive equation in the critically ill since this equation is based on healthy individuals and has not been well researched in the critically ill.

Box 1
Predictive equations

Harris-Benedict-not recommended for critical care patients

Men = 66.4730 + (13.7516 × weight) + (5.0033 × height) − (6.7550 × age)

Women = 655.0955 + (9.5634 × weight) + (1.8496 × height) − (4.6756 × age)

1992 Ireton-Jones-recommended for both non-obese or obese critical care patients

1,925 − (10 × age) + (5 × weight) + (281 if male) + (292 if trauma present) + (851 if burns present)

1998 Penn State-recommended for critical care obese patients

(1.1 × value from Harris-Benedict equation[a]) + (140 × T_{max}) + (32 × V_E) − 5,340

2003 Penn State-recommended for critical care non-obese patients

(0.85 × value from Harris-Benedict equation[b]) + (175 × T_{max}) + (33 × V_E) − 6,433

Swinamer-recommended for critical care nonobese patients

(945 × BSA) − (6.4 × age) + (108 × temperature) + (24.2 × RR) + (817 × V_T) − 4,349

Weight in kilograms, height in centimeters, age in years.
Abbreviations: BSA, body surface area (m^2); T_{max}, max body temperature in Celsius for past 24 hours; RR, respiratory rate in breaths per minute; V_E, minute volume (L/min); V_T, tidal volume (L).
    [a] Use adjusted body weight with obese patients (add 25% of excess body weight to ideal body weight).
    [b] Use actual body weight.

NURSING DIAGNOSIS

After all data has been collected regarding the patient's nutritional state and needs, a plan of care can be formulated based on nursing diagnoses identified for the patient. The purpose of developing a plan of care is to communicate with other nurses and health care team members and to provide direction for the care of the patient. It also assists with evaluating how accurate assessment, diagnoses, planning, implementation and evaluation are when providing patient care to the patient.[25]

PLANNING

During the planning stage, the nurse assigns priorities to the identified nursing diagnoses; priority is given to the problems that are most urgent and critical. Goals and expected outcomes are derived from the diagnoses. They can be assigned as short, intermediate, or long-term and they should be specific, measurable and patient-focused with an identified time frame for achievement.[18]

Goals for nutrition therapy in critically ill patients are to lessen the metabolic response to stress, prevent oxidative cellular injury, and promote favorable modulation of the immune response through "early enteral nutrition, appropriate macro- and micronutritent delivery and meticulous glycemic control,"[13] Proactively providing early nutrition support can support these goals, which in turn reduces disease severity, diminishes complications, decreases ICU length of stay and promotes favorable outcomes for patients.[13]

Critical care patients should receive enough calories to support anabolic function, while excess calories should be avoided. Recommendations are for 25 kcal/kg of usual body weight per day for the majority of patients. In obese patients who have a BMI > 25 kg/m^2, ideal body weight should be used in calculation. Patients who have a BMI > 30 kg/m^2 should receive between 60% to 70% of energy requirements or 11–14 kcal/kg actual weight or 22–25 kcal/kg ideal body weight per day.[13] For patients with a BMI < 16 kg/m^2, actual body weight should be calculated for the first 7 to10 days and then ideal body weight should be used.[24] Any additional calories that the patient may be receiving including lipids from infusions such as Propofol should be included.[13]

Research has shown meeting protein requirements in the critically ill can improve morbidity and mortality. Protein recommendations are 1.5–2.0 g/kg or 20%–25% of total calories from protein for most postoperative critically ill patients, with the exception of renal or hepatic insufficiency patients being on protein restrictions.[27] Critical care patients with a BMI < 30 kg/m^2 need between 1.2–2.0 g/kg of protein per actual body weight per day. Other critically ill patients, such as multiple trauma and burn patients, will likely need higher protein requirements. For critically ill obese patients with a BMI of 30–40 kg/m^2, protein recommendations are for $\geq$ 2.0 g/kg ideal body weight per day. For patients with a BMI $\geq$ 40 kg/m^2 provide $\geq$ 2.5 g/kg protein daily.[13] The goal is to achieve a net protein anabolism.[10]

Immune-modulating enteral formulas should be considered in patients with head and neck cancer, less than 30% total body surface area burns, less than 20 abdominal trauma index score, and patients undergoing major gastrointestinal surgery along with non-severely septic mechanically ventilated patients.[26] Unlike traditional enteral formulas, immune-modulating formulas include any combination of arginine, glutamine, nucleic acid, n-3 fatty acids, and antioxidants. Five meta-analyses have found immune-modulating formulas linked to significant reductions in patient length of stay, mechanical ventilation days, and infectious morbidity.[13] Heyland and colleagues[28–31] concluded in a systematic review with a subgroup of critically ill patients that immunonutrition was consistent with a reduction in length of stay, but it had no overall impact on patient mortality or rate of infectious complications.

The ADA[15] does not recommend routine use of immune-enhancing enteral nutrition for trauma or critically ill patients as its use may also be associated with increased mortality in the severely ill critical care population. The Canadian Clinical Practice Guidelines (2009) do not recommend diets supplemented with arginine and other select nutrients for all critical care patients, but they do suggest the use of antioxidant vitamins and trace minerals for critically ill patients.[26] SCCM/ASPEN Guidelines (2009) support the use of antioxidant vitamins and trace minerals in all critical care patients receiving nutritional therapy.[13]

In acute respiratory distress syndrome and severe acute lung injury patients immune-modulating enteral formula with an anti-inflammatory lipid profile containing fish oils, borage oils, and antioxidants are recommended.[13,26] This formula was found to significantly reduce length of stay in critical care, mechanical ventilation time, organ failure, and mortality versus use of standard formulation.

Selecting the best formula for each critical care patient can be a challenge as a large number of enteral formulations are commercially available. High-lipid, low carbohydrate and calorically-dense fluid restricted enteral formulas should be used for acute respiratory failure patients. Standard enteral formulas should be used for acute renal failure or acute kidney injury patients without significant electrolyte abnormalities, but for patients on hemodialysis or continuous renal replacement therapy, an enhanced protein formulation, up to 2.5 g/kg/d should be provided.[13]

Acute and chronic liver patients should receive standard enteral formulas, while branched chain amino acid formulations should be considered in patients with hepatic encephalopathy refractory to typical treatment. Small peptide and medium-chain triglyeride or almost fat-free elemental enteral formulations are worthy of consideration in patients with severe acute pancreatitis.[13]

Providing enteral nutrition to a critically ill obese patient requires the placement of an enteral feeding device. Which tube to use and how to place it should be a part of the planning stage. It is the purpose of this article to primarily cover those tubes that can be placed by a nurse. There is very little data available to identify whether a specific type of tube or placement technique can be of benefit to obese critically ill patients, except in those patients that have undergone bariatric surgery. For those patients, it is advisable to consult with a physician for tube placement.

Enteral feeding tubes are usually placed nasally or orally and are for short-term access. Tubes can be placed blindly or with assistance of specialized equipment and techniques. Large bore tubes such as a NG tube can only be placed into the stomach. Small bore tubes can be placed with the distal tip either in the stomach or advanced into the small bowel.

Some patients will require the use of a tube for longer periods of time than others. This need may or may not be immediately apparent. There are long-term tube options for these patients such as gastrostomy, jejunostomy, percutaneous endoscopic gastrostomy (PEG), percutaneous endoscopic jejunostomy (PEJ) and percutanous endoscopic gastrostomy jejunostomy (PEGJ) tubes. All of these tubes require placement by a surgeon or specially trained physician. They also have associated complications including procedural related mishaps, site infection, leakage, buried bumper syndrome, tube malfunction and inadvertent removal.[32]

Tubes that are placed nasally can incur epistaxis during the placement procedure or sinusitis as a long-term consequence.[32] However, some patients may not be able to tolerate a tube being present orally, particularly if they are alert and aware. Patient comfort and the situation should be considered when choosing which orifice will be used to introduce the feeding tube.

Large bore feeding tubes have some advantages in that they provide the nurse the ability to evaluate residual feeding volumes in the patient's stomach and the tube is less prone to becoming occluded. In their study of 60 ICU patients, Neumann and deLegge[33] found that patients who had their tubes placed in the stomach received their feeding with fewer placement attempts, were fed more quickly, and achieved their goal rate sooner than those whose tubes were placed post-pylorically. If the patient does not have a NG tube that can be used appropriately, a decision will need to be made regarding the type of tube, the route of placement, and location for the distal end of the tube.

If a tube is placed blindly, there are a number of techniques that can assist the nurse to ensure that the tube is not inadvertently placed into the tracheobronchial tree, which can occur in two to four percent of placements.[34] These techniques include: observing for signs of respiratory distress or inability to speak, measuring pH of fluid withdrawn, auscultation of air insufflated through the tube, and observing for bubbling when the end of the tube is held underwater.[35] Devices that can assist during the placement process include colorimetric carbon dioxide detectors, capnography, magnetically guided feeding tube, and electromagnetic tube feeding placement device.[34]

Colorimetric carbon dioxide detectors are attached to the feeding tube after the tube has been placed to detect the presence of carbon dioxide. Tubes that have been placed into the tracheobronchial tree will visually display the presence of carbon dioxide by a color change in the detector and should be removed and replaced enterally. Capnography has also been used during the placement process for the same reason but requires specialized equipment to do this.[34]

There is no sure nonradiographic method to differentiate whether the tube has been placed in the respiratory tract, esophagus, stomach or small bowel.[35] Because none of these above described methods are confirmatory, it is imperative to radiographically confirm the placement of the tube before feeding the patient.[36] The length of the tube that is outside the patient should be marked and carefully monitored at regular intervals. Tubes that have been dislodged should be re-evaluated and confirmed by radiograph before feedings are continued.[36]

Some critically ill patients may not be able to tolerate enteral feedings into the stomach. The problem is often caused by issues of impaired gastric motility, decreased level of consciousness, or strict supine positioning, which place the patient at greater risk for regurgitation and aspiration.[26] Inotropes, continuous infusion of opioids, sedatives, or paralytics can interfere with gastric motility. For these patients, providing feedings postpylorically minimizes risk of aspiration while providing the patient with needed nutrients in a safe and effective manner.[20] When tubes are placed postpylorically, it is recommended that the tube be advanced to past the ligament of Treitz to reduce the possibility of aspiration from feeding regurgitating from the small bowel into the stomach.[34]

Placement of enteral feeding devices postpylorically can be more difficult and may delay the start of enteral nutrition while placement is attempted.[20] To reduce this delay, practitioners have historically used fluoroscopy or endoscopy to ensure post-pyloric tube placement, but these are costly and also usually require transport of the patient to a procedure area that may not be within the confines of the critical care environment, which places the patient at risk for untoward events associated with transportation.[37]

In the oldest of three meta-analyses comparing NG to postpyloric or small bowel feeding comparing 612 patients, there was a significant reduction in ventilator associated pneumonia (VAP) without a significant reduction in mortality for patients who were fed postpylorically.[26] In the subsequent two meta-analyses with a combined population of 1159 patients, there was no difference in occurrence of pneumonia or length of ICU stay. It was also found that patients fed by gastric route were fed sooner than those patients whose tubes were placed postpylorically.[38,39] Currently, the recommendation is to use the gastric route unless the patient has specific reason for placement of feeding past the stomach.[13]

Newer devices are available on the market that can assist the nurse at the bedside to place tubes postpylorically. The magnetic guided feeding tube (MGFT) has a magnet at its distal end and a magnetic field sensor. The sensor is connected to a light indicator at its proximal end. A handheld external magnet is placed over the abdomen and moved in a specified manner to maneuver and steer the tube tip through the pylorus into the duodenum. Published rates of success range from 60% to 88% on the first try, with an average procedure time of just 15 minutes.[34]

The electronic tube placement device (ETPD) can also assist the nurse at the bedside to place the feeding tube into the small bowel. A small electronic device is placed over the patient's xyphoid process and is able to display onto a computer screen the location of the distal tip of the feeding tube, which has an electronic sensor. Published rates of success range up to 90% to 100%, with average time to placement in under 15 minutes using ETPD.[34]

Both the MGFT and ETPD have been proven to be effective and efficient, but they do cost additional money for purchase of equipment, special feeding tubes and training for nurses to be able to use them correctly both initially and through ongoing competency assessment. This additional cost must be weighed against the costs of delayed nutrition, nursing time, number of tube placements that it can potentially be used for, aspiration and VAP prevention and even potential costs of a sentinel event from feeding being inadvertently routed into the tracheobronchial tree. Use of this equipment can also improve patient comfort and nurse satisfaction from reduced time to placement.

If MGFT and ETPD are not available there are techniques and medications that can be used at the bedside to help assist the nurse to efficiently place feeding tubes postpylorically.[20] Use of promotility agents, such as erythromycin and metoclopramide, can assist with movement of blindly placed enteral tubes postpylorically and metoclopromide has the added benefit of improving gastrointestinal transit and feeding tolerance.[40] Although effective the techniques do require training to learn and are generally more time-consuming than the above described specialized equipment. Increased practice can improve the time needed to achieve successful placement using these techniques with or without the use of promotility agents.

Safety is of utmost concern for all patients and safe choices should be practiced routinely. Standardized labels should be used that identify patient, formula, route, hang date/time and individual hanging formula.[36] All enteral feeding components should clearly state that they are not for intravenous use and connectors should only operate with enteral access components. Only oral syringes that can be used with enteral components should be used to administer medications into the enteral feeding system.[36]

IMPLEMENTATION

During the implementation stage, the activities of the health care team, patient and family are coordinated. Interventions can be provided by the nurse or, if appropriate, can be delegated to other health care providers or to patient or family members. It is important to document the patient's responses to care provided.[18]

Research has shown that using feeding protocols that are nurse-driven can improve the percentage of goal calories delivered to patients. All enteral nutrition orders should have patient identifiers, the formula ordered, enteral access delivery site/device, and the administration method and rate.[36] Protocols should address the goal rate of the infusion, orders for managing gastric residual volumes (GRV), frequency of flushes, and conditions or problems under which feeding may be adjusted or stopped.[13]

In the implementation stage, feeding delivery to the patient is begun. Rates of feeding as low as 10–30 mL per hour can prevent mucosal atrophy and protect the immune function of the gut, but these rates are not enough to achieve the results of providing enteral therapy at the goal rate that is required to meet the patient's metabolic demands for nutrition.[13] Providing nutrition at rates at more than 50% to 65% of the patient's targeted goal during the first week of hospitalization can improve clinical outcomes.[13]

Feeding pumps with hourly rate increases of 10–20 mL/hour every 8 to 12 hours are preferred for critically ill patients. Achievement of the goal rate should occur within 48 to 72 hours. If the goal rate cannot be achieved within 7 to 10 days, parenteral nutrition should be considered.[13]

Back-rest elevation can be raised from 30° to 45° while the patient is supine to reduce the risk of aspiration and VAP. If the patient is unable to tolerate hip flexion, a reverse Trendelenberg can be used to achieve head elevation.[13] Oral hygiene can also assist in the prevention of VAP: adding a chlorhexidine mouthwash twice a day to oral care routines has been shown to prevent nosocomial respiratory infections.[13]

Residual volumes are often a concern in the critical care patient because of the potential for regurgitation and aspiration. Traditionally, feedings have been withheld for lack of bowel sounds, presence of residual volumes > 200 mL, or diarrhea. None of these are evidence-based practices and they result in undernourishment of patients.[9] Blue food coloring should never be added to enteral feedings to evaluate for aspiration as this has been shown to be harmful to patients.[13]

Risk factors for aspiration include: presence of nasoenteric tube, endotracheal tube with mechanical ventilation, age > 70 years, increased nurse patient ratios, patient position, transport out of the ICU, and use of bolus intermittent feedings.[13]

To accurately evaluate GRV, the patient should have a large bore feeding tube in place. GRV can be checked to evaluate the amount of fluids in the stomach every 4 hours for the first 48 hours.[13] This procedure cannot consistently be done accurately with small bore feeding tubes. If GRV is ≥ 250 mL after a second check, the use of a promotility agents should be considered.[13] Metoclopramide is preferred over erythromycin,[26] but some protocols call for the use of both.[13] Hold feedings for repeat GRV > 500 mL and consider placing the feeding tube in the post-pyloric position because this change can improve nutritional delivery to these patients and reduce the risk of regurgitation and aspiration.[26]

Withholding feedings for high GRV is usually accompanied by additional signs of feeding intolerance, such as patient complaint of pain and or distention, physical examination, absence of flatus and or stool, and abdominal radiographs.[13] Feedings do not need to be stopped for brief periods of backrest recline during nursing procedures, such as linen changes, because delays in restarting feeding can occur also interfering with total nutrition delivered. Feedings should be held for procedures that require head of bed to be below 30° for prolonged periods of time or for known repeat high gastric residuals.[13]

Diarrhea is also a concern that may be present with some patients. Assess the patient for excessive intake of hyperosmolar medications such as sorbitol (a commonly used substance in liquid medications), use of broad spectrum antibiotics, presence of Clostridium difficile, pseudomembranous colitis, or other infectious problems.[13]

If diarrhea is present and causative agents have been eliminated, use of formulas that have soluble fiber or small peptide formulations can be helpful.[13] However, there is not enough data to support the routine use of these formulas for all critically ill patients.[26] Insoluble fiber should be avoided.[13]

The nurse can do much to prevent nosocomial infection in critically ill patients through maintaining clean technique when handling the feeding system, taking care not to introduce pathogens. Use of closed systems is helpful as formula can be hung for 24–48 hours. Formula in open systems should hang for no more than 8 hours, or 4 hours if it is powdered or reconstituted.[36] Tap water should not be used for hydration or flushes, diluting medications or formula reconstitution as its use has been shown to cause infection in patients. Use sterile or distilled water instead.[36]

If oral versions are not available, dilute each medication to be administered with at least 30 mL water and administer each separately with 15 mL water given between. This process can reduce the risk of tube clogging because some medications do interact with one another to form precipitates that can cause clogging.[36] Consideration should be given to the amount of fluid that is being given during medication administration because this will have an effect on patient's overall fluid balance.

Flushing regularly with 30 mL of water every 4 hours and after medication administration through the feeding tube helps to maintain patency of the tube. Water is superior to cranberry juice or carbonated beverages to maintain patency.[36] Pancrelipase and sodium bicarbonate may be helpful in re-establishing patency of clogged tubes.[36]

Probiotics can also be helpful for critically ill patients that have received a transplant, major abdominal surgery, or severe trauma.[13] However, routine use of prebiotics, synbiotics and probiotics cannot be recommended for all critically ill patients because there is not enough evidence to support their use.[26]

Opioids are commonly used to ensure comfort of critically ill patients, but these drugs can also reduce gastric motility and result in constipation. Administering 8 mg of naloxone enterally every 6 hours was found to counter these effects and to increase the amount of feeding delivered, reduce gastric volumes, and decrease the incidence of VAP in one study.[41]

EVALUATION

During the evaluation stage, the nurse determines the success of the plan of care and if there is a need to alter it. This decision requires careful assessment of data collected and documented during the implementation stage comparing the patient's actual outcomes to expected outcomes. If alterations are required they should be evidence-based and reflect the individualized needs of the patient. Because the nursing process is cyclical, newly added or altered interventions should again be assessed in regard to whether they meet the patient's needs and assist with improving outcomes.[18]

The nurse cannot depend on one single indicator for presence or degree of malnutrition.[4] There are many factors that should be considered when determining whether the patient's nutritional needs are being met. Actual enteral intake should be evaluated daily when monitoring critically ill patients.[15] If intake is less than the requirements, a nurse should explore the reasons for this result and take corrective action.

Monitoring of daily weight is a common practice in the critical care setting. Although weight itself is not diagnostic, it a can be used in a gross assessment of a patient's nutritional status. However, in a critically ill obese patient, weight loss may be therapeutic. Permissive underfeeding is a way to help the patient to achieve weight loss, increase insulin sensitivity in some patients, improve the ability of nurses to provide care, and reduce the risk of some comorbidities.[13]

Weight losses and gains should be considered in light of the patient's overall fluid balance. In critically ill patients, weight changes may be more reflective of edema and volume overload than true body cell mass.[24] If IC is available, patients can be serially monitored for the REE and RQ to determine if the nutrition delivered is meeting the metabolic demands of the patients.[22]

In their study of 40 critically ill obese patients, Dickerson and colleagues found that hypocaloric feedings of < 20 kcal/kg/day significantly reduced ICU length of stay and duration of antibiotic therapy. There was a trend toward reduction in ventilator days in the treatment group. All patients received at least 2 g/kg/day protein in their feedings.[12,42]

Laboratory values can also be monitored to identify if nutritional needs are being met. Albumin levels of < 35 g/L in acutely ill patients indicates catabolism and decreased stores of amino acids. In addition, they indicate prolonged physiologic stress and can prolong ventilator weaning.[43] Pre-albumin has a shorter half-life of 3 days and can be a more immediate indicator of protein stores and usage, but its levels can be falsely elevated if the patient is receiving steroids or is on dialysis.[4]

Excessive hypoalbuminemia reduces colloid osmotic pressure, which can, in turn, cause fluid overload resulting in renal failure, cardiac failure and death, as is seen in refeeding syndrome.[17] To monitor for this deadly phenomenon, electrolytes and glucose levels should also be monitored at least daily and more often if needed.[4]

Both hyperglycemia and hypoglycemia should be avoided in all critically ill patients as both have deleterious effects. The exact range at which glucose should be maintained is still controversial and undecided, but most recent evidence suggests that levels should be maintained < 140–150 mg/dL.[44] Glucose levels most likely should be maintained at 80–110 mg/dL in critically ill surgical patients as opposed to all other critically ill patients because tight glycemic control has been shown to be of distinct benefit to this population.[13,45]

Electrolytes should be maintained in normal ranges to prevent refeeding syndrome or other associated complications,[16] particularly magnesium and phosphorus levels, which play an important role in energy synthesis and wound healing.[43] Hemoglobin can also indicate nutritional state and is important in the ability of the blood to carry oxygen so levels should be regularly monitored.[43]

In addition to albumin and pre-albumin, total lymphocyte count, transferrin and retinol binding iron measurements, and urine creatinine clearance are often measured to evaluate the patient's nutritional state, but none of these are accurate measurements in the critically ill patient as they are all altered by increases in vascular permeability and reprioritization of hepatic protein synthesis that occur during critical illness.[4,13]

Protein overfeeding can be evaluated by BUN that is stable in relation to creatinine levels. Fat overload is measured by increasing triglycerides of > 500 mg/dL.[4] Overfeeding should be avoided because it results in excessive carbon dioxide production, which can increase the work of breathing and impair ventilator weaning.[2]

Finally, the patient's hydration status should be evaluated by physical assessment, such as appearance of skin and mucous membranes. Monitor fluid balance and lab values, such as sodium, BUN and creatinine closely.[4]

SUMMARY

The nursing process provides the framework for meeting the nutritional needs of critically ill obese patients. It is well known that early enteral feeding can be of great benefit to patients who have an intact gastrointestinal tract because it can reduce the complications from infections and length of stay in critically ill patients.[39]

Caring for obese critically ill patients is not always the same as caring for critically ill patients who are not obese. Fortunately, nurses have many resources available to them to guide them in this process. However, research that specifically addresses the needs of obese critically ill patients is still lacking in many areas and should be considered as potential areas to develop evidence-based practices.

When there is a lack of data to support practice applications specific to obese patients, it is up to the clinician to consider the individual patient's state and to evaluate effectiveness of care delivered during the cyclical nursing process. A variety of guidelines are available to the bedside practitioner, but they are not universally used.

Barriers exist within every ICU to implementation of evidence-based practices.[28,46] Achieving excellent outcomes entails efforts to bring evidence-based practices to the patient in the bed. Critical care nurses can be instrumental in advocating for their patients and ensuring that the care patients receive is standard of practice and individualized to their needs using the nursing process.

REFERENCES

1. Ogden CL, Carroll MD, Curtin LR, et al. Prevalence of overweight and obesity in the United States, 1999–2004. JAMA 2006;295(13):1549–55.
2. Dickerson RN. Hypocaloric feeding of obese patients in the intensive care unit. Curr Opin Clin Nutr Metab Care 2005;8:189–96.
3. Brown B, Turek J, Maillet JO. Comparison of an institutional nutrition screen with 4 validated nutrition screening tools. Top Clin Nutr 2006;21(2):122–38.
4. Harrington L. Nutrition in critically ill adults: key process and outcomes. Crit Care Nurs Clin North Am 2004;16(2004):459–65.
5. Zaloga GP. Parenteral nutrition in adult patients with functioning gastrointestinal tracts: assessment of outcomes. Lancet 2006;367:1101–11.
6. Zizza C, Herring AH, Stevens J, et al. Length of hospital stay among obese individuals. Am J Public Health 2005;94(9):1587–91.
7. Joffe A, Wood K. Obesity in critical care. Curr Opin Anaesthesiol 2007;20:113–8.
8. Akinnusi ME, Pineda LA, Solh AA. Effect of obesity on intensive care morbidity and mortality: a meta-analysis. Crit Care Med 2008;36(1):151–8.
9. Swanson RW, Winkleman C. Special feature: exploring the benefits and myths of enteral feeding in the critically ill. Crit Care Nurs Q 2002;24(4):67–74.
10. Elamin EM. Nutritional care of the obese intensive care unit patient. Curr Opin Crit Care 2005;11:300–3.
11. World Health Organization (1995, 2000, 2004). BMI classification. Available at: http://apps.who.int/bmi/index.jsp?introPage=intro_3.html. Accessed on July 7, 2009.
12. Anonymous. Life cycle and metabolic conditions. J Parenter Eternal Nutr 2002; 27(1):SA45–59.
13. McClave SA, Martindale RG, Vanek VW, et al. Guidelines for the provision of assessment of nutrition support therapy in the adult critically ill patient: Society of Critical Care Medicine (S.C.C.M.) and American Society for Parenteral and Enteral Nutrition (A.S.P.E.N. J Parenter Enteral Nutr 2009;33(3):277–316.

14. Choban PS, Dickerson RN. Morbid obesity and nutrition support: is bigger different? Nutr Clin Pract 2005;20:480–7.
15. American Dietetic Association. Critical illness evidence-based nutrition practice guideline. Chicago: American Dietetic Association; 2006. Available at: http://www.adaevidencelibrary.com/topic.cfm?cat=3016. Accessed on July 5, 2009.
16. Adkins SM. Recognizing and preventing refeeding syndrome. Dimens Crit Care Nurs 2009;28(2):53–8.
17. Flesher ME, Archer KA, Leslie BD, et al. Assessing the metabolic and clinical consequences of early enteral feeding in the malnourished patient. J Parenter Enteral Nutr 2005;29(2):108–17.
18. Nettina SM, editor. Lippincott manual of nursing practice. 9th edition. Philadelphia: Lippincott, Williams and Wilkins; 2009.
19. Doig GS, Simpson F, Finfer F, et al. Nutrition Guidelines Investigators of the ANZICS Clinical Trials Group. JAMA 2008;300(23):2731–41.
20. Powers J, Chance R, Bortenschlager L, et al. Bedside placement of small-bowel feeding tubes in the intensive care unit. Crit Care Nurse 2003;23(1):16–23.
21. Frankenfeld D, Hise M, Malone A, et al. Prediction of resting metabolic rate in critically ill adult patients: results of a systematic review of the evidence. Journal of the American Dietetic Association 2007;107(9):1552–61.
22. Haugen HA, Chan LN, Li F. Indirect calorimetry: a practical guide for clinicians. Nutr Clin Pract 2007;22(4):377–88.
23. Fujii TK, Phillips BJ. Quick review: the metabolic cart. J Intern Med 2003;3(2). Available at: http://www.ispub.com/journal/the_internet_journal_of_internal_medicine/volume_3_number_2_25/article/quick_review_the_metabolic_cart.html. Accessed on July 6, 2009.
24. Walker RN, Heuberger RA. Predictive equations for energy needs for the critically ill. Respir Care 2009;54(4):509–21.
25. Carpenito-Moyet LJ. Nursing care plans and documentation: nursing diagnoses and collaborative problems. Philadelphia: Lippincott, Williams and Wilkins; 2009.
26. Heyland DK, Dhaliwal R, Drover DW, et al. Guidelines Committee. Canadian clinical practice guidelines for nutrition support in adult critically ill patients. J Parenter Eternal Nutr 2003;27(5):355–73 Updated recommendations 2007 and 2009. Available at: http://www.criticalcarenutrition.com/docs/cpg/srrev.pdf Accessed on July 5, 2009.
27. Ventura JM. Protein requirements and losses: Surgical wounds and drains. Support Line. 2008;30(6):8–13.
28. Heyland DK, Noval F, Drover JW, et al. Should immunonutrients become routine in critically ill patients? A systematic review of the evidence. JAMA 2001;286(8):944–53.
29. Heyland DK, Drover JW, Dhaliwal R, et al. Optimizing the benefits and minimizing the risks of enteral nutrition in the critically ill: Role of small bowel feeding. J Parenter Enteral Nutr 2002;26(6):S51–7.
30. McCowen KC, Bistrian BR. Immunonutrition: problematic or problem solving? Am J Clin Nutr 2003;77:764–70.
31. Adams GF, Guest DP, Ciraulo DL, et al. Maximizing tolerance of enteral nutrition in severely injured trauma patients: a comparison of enteral feedings by means of percutaneous endoscopic versus percutaneous endoscopic gastrojejunostomy. J Trauma 2000;48(3):459–65.
32. Baskin WN. Acute complications associated with bedside placement of feeding tubes. Nutrition in Clinical Practice 2006;21(1):40–55.

33. Neumann DA, DeLegge MH. Gastric versus small-bowel tube feeding in the intensive care unit: a prospective comparison of efficacy. Crit Care Med 2002; 30(7):1436–8.

34. Roberts S, Echeverria P, Gabriel S. Devices and techniques for bedside enteral feeding tube placement. Nutrition in Clinical Practice 2007;22(4):412–20.

35. Metheny NA, Meert KL. Monitoring feeding tube placement. Nutrition in Clinical Practice 2004;19(5):487–95.

36. Bankhead R, Boullata J, Corkins M, et al. ASPEN enteral nutrition practice recommendations. J Parenter Eternal Nutr 2009;33(2):122–67.

37. Searley HE. Patients' outcomes: intrahospital transport and monitoring of critically ill patients by a specially trained ICU nursing staff. Am J Crit Care 1998;7(4):282–7.

38. Ho KM, Dobb GJ, Webb SA. A comparison of early gastric and post-pyloric feeding in critically ill patients: a meta-analysis. Intensive Care Med 2006;32(5): 639–49.

39. Marik PE, Zaloga GP. Early enteral nutrition in acutely ill patients: a systematic review. Crit Care Med 2001;29(12):2264–70.

40. Booth CM, Heyland DK, Paterson WG. Gastrointestinal promotility drugs in the critical care setting: a systematic review of the evidence. Crit Care Med 2002; 30(7):1429–35.

41. Meissner W, Dohrn B, Reinhart K. Enteral naloxone reduces gastric tube reflux and frequency of pneumonia in critical care patients during opioid analgesia. Crit Care Med 2003;31(3):776–80.

42. Dickerson RN, Boschert KJ, Kudsk KA, et al. Hypocaloric enteral tube feeding in critically ill obese patients. Nutrition 2002;18(3):241–6.

43. Higgins PA, Daly BJ, Lipson AR, et al. Assessing nutritional status in chronically critically ill adult patients. Am J Crit Care 2006;15(2):166–77.

44. Fahy BG, Sheehy AM, Coursin DM. Glucose control in the intensive care unit. Crit Care Med 2009;37(5):1769–76.

45. Griesdale DEG, de Souza RJ, van Dam RM, et al. Intensive insulin therapy and mortality among critically ill patients: a meta-analysis including NICE-SUGAR study data. Can Med Assoc J 2008;180(8):821–7.

46. Jones NE, Heyland DK. Implementing nutrition guidelines in the critical care setting: is it a worthwhile and achievable goal? JAMA 2008;300(23):2798–9.

Impact of Obesity on Care of Postoperative Coronary Bypass Patients

Barbara Leeper, MN, RN, CNS, CCRN

KEYWORDS

- Coronary artery bypass graft surgery • CABG
- Morbid obesity • Cardiac surgery • Obesity

Obesity has become a major health problem in the United States and is well known to be a risk factor for the development of cardiovascular disease. There are an estimated 97 million overweight or obese adults (67% of adults) in the United States, which has increased by 50% since the 1960s.[1] Recent data from the American Heart Association indicate among normal-weight white adults between the ages of 30 and 59 years, the 4-year rate of becoming overweight (body mass index ≥ 25 kg/m^2) increased from 14% to 19% in females and from 26% to 30% in males.[2] One in 10 individuals was found to have a body mass index (BMI) equal to or greater than 35 kg/m^2 across different age groups.[2] (Refer to **Table 1** for definitions of BMI and weight descriptions.) The rate of extreme obesity has increased from 4.7% of individuals to 5.9%, with some states reporting an incidence as high as 19.3% (Colorado) and 32.6% (Mississippi).[2] The direct cost of obesity is estimated to be $56.1 billion; 17% or $6.99 billion can be attributed to cardiac costs.[1]

Many clinicians perceive obesity, particularly severe or morbid obesity, to be associated with increased risk for mortality and morbidity. This article reviews the literature addressing the risk for morbidity and mortality associated with obese patients undergoing coronary artery bypass graft (CABG) surgery. Implications for nursing practice are addressed with recommendations for practice in this patient population.

OBESITY AND SURGICAL MORTALITY RISK

There have been many studies examining the risks of CABG surgery in the obese patient population. Most have concluded that CABG surgery is safe in this group of individuals.

Cardiovascular Services, Baylor University Medical Center, 3500 Gaston Avenue, Dallas, TX 75246, USA
E-mail address: bobbi.leeper@baylorhealth.edu

Crit Care Nurs Clin N Am 21 (2009) 369–375
doi:10.1016/j.ccell.2009.07.003
0899-5885/09/$ – see front matter © 2009 Elsevier Inc. All rights reserved.
ccnursing.theclinics.com

Table 1
Classification of body mass index

Body Mass Index	Description
<18.5 kg/m²	Underweight
18.5–25.9 kg/m²	Normal weight
≥30 kg/m²	Obesity
>40.0 kg/m²	Extreme obesity

Data from Refs.[1,2,7]

One of the first large studies investigating obesity and the risk for adverse outcomes associated with CABG surgery was conducted by the Northern New England Cardiovascular Disease Study Group in 1998.[3] They analyzed 11,101 consecutive patients who had CABG surgery between 1992 and 1996. Patients were classified, based on BMI, into quartiles, with non-obesity defined as BMI 30 kg/m² or less, obesity BMI 31 to 36 kg/m², and severe obesity BMI greater than 36 kg/m². They assessed the independent contribution of obesity to postoperative outcomes, including in-hospital mortality, stroke, postoperative bleeding, and sternal wound infections associated with CABG surgery. Their findings demonstrated obesity was not associated with increased mortality or postoperative stroke. Obesity and severe obesity were associated with increased risk for sternal wound infection (obesity: adjusted odds ratio [OR], 2.10; CI, 1.45–3.06; $P<.001$; severe obesity: adjusted OR, 2.74; CI, 1.49–5.02; $P = .001$). Postoperative bleeding rates were significantly lower in both groups.[3]

Brandt and colleagues[4] studied 500 consecutive patients undergoing CABG surgery. There were 100 severely obese (BMI > 30 kg/m²) patients in the group. The severely obese patients were slightly younger and had hypertension and diabetes. No significant differences were observed between the two groups related to morbidity and mortality.

In 2002, there were several published studies addressing the risk for morbidity and mortality in obese patients having CABG. Prabhakar and colleagues[1] used the Society of Thoracic Surgeons (STS) National Cardiac Database to investigate the independent effect of moderate obesity (BMI 35–39.9 kg/m²) and extreme obesity (BMI ≥ 40 kg/m²) on CABG surgery outcomes. A total of 559,000 patients underwent first-time CABG surgery between January 1997 and December 2000 and served as the basis for this study. The observational analysis of study findings indicated moderately obese patients had slightly elevated operative risk (adjusted OR, 1.21; CI, 1.13–1.29). Extremely obese patients had significantly higher risk for operative mortality (OR, 1.58; CI, 1.45–1.73). The investigators found the extremely obese patients had more major postoperative complications, including deep sternal wound infections, renal failure, and prolonged hospital length of stay. Although the investigators concluded that extreme obesity (BMI ≥ 40 kg/m²) is a significant predictor for adverse outcomes and increased hospital length of stay, they stated a limitation of this study was using patients from the STS database, which may not represent the general population because not all cardiac surgery programs participate in the STS database.[1]

Maurer and colleagues[5] studied 1148 patients aged 75 years and older who underwent cardiac surgery between 1991 and 1999. Patients were divided into tertiles, with a BMI less than 25 kg/m² defined as normal, BMI greater than 25 kg/m² defined as overweight, and BMI greater than 30 kg/m² defined as obese. Their results indicated that geriatric patients who had lower BMI (<23 kg/m²) had a higher risk for complications, including stroke, bleeding, respiratory failure, ventricular arrhythmias, and mortality, than those who had higher BMI. They did not find that higher BMI was associated with increased risk for complications, excluding wound infections.[5]

Another group conducted a retrospective study of 4713 consecutive patients undergoing CABG surgical procedures. Their purpose was to examine the relationship between obesity and in-hospital outcomes. There were 1041 non-obese (BMI < 30 kg/m^2) patients compared with 1041 obese (BMI 30–35 kg/m^2) and 23 severely obese (BMI > 35 kg/m^2) patients. These researchers did not find any association between obesity and in-hospital mortality, stroke, myocardial infarction, reoperation for bleeding, or renal failure. They did find an association between obesity and the incidence of atrial arrhythmias and sternal wound infections.[6]

Jin and coworkers[7] studied 16,232 patients who underwent CABG surgery at nine Providence Health System hospitals in the northwest. Using a logistical regression model, these researchers found body size was not a risk factor for increased mortality. They found the lowest mortality to be in those patients in the high-normal and overweight body groups (OR 0.61 (0.47–0.80); CI .95).[7] Subsequent studies have reported similar findings.[8–14]

Most of these studies demonstrated morbidly obese patients undergoing CABG surgery do not have an increased mortality risk. The number of patients studied is certainly significant. Several of the studies use different definitions for overweight, obesity, and severe obesity, which is a limiting factor. Three reported higher mortality rates in underweight people.[1,8,9] Investigators did comment that when compared with those patients who had a normal BMI, the severely and morbidly obese patients were much younger and had diabetes and hypertension.

OBESITY AND MORBIDITY
Impact of Diabetes

The morbidity and mortality associated with the metabolic syndrome is well known, and therefore is considered to be a major risk factor for negative outcomes.[15] Some believe that the obese patient who has diabetes may be at risk for systemic proinflammatory and thrombotic states, which contribute to poorer postoperative outcomes following CABG surgery. Pan and coworkers[16] conducted a retrospective study of patients (n = 9862) who underwent primary CABG surgery between 1995 and 2004. Their results did not indicate that obese patients who had diabetes were at higher risk for adverse postoperative complications, including death, stroke, myocardial infarction, sepsis, and sternal wound infection. They did find that obesity in a patient who had diabetes was independently associated with a significantly increased risk for respiratory failure postoperatively (OR, 2.26; 95% CI, 1.41–3.61; $P<.001$), along with atrial fibrillation, ventricular tachycardia, and leg wound infections.

Of interest is a study conducted by Shah and colleagues.[17] These investigators studied the effect of metabolic syndrome on survival in patients who had established coronary artery disease. The patient population included patients undergoing revascularization therapy, both catheter-based procedures and CABG surgery. The study sample included 2886 patients who had confirmed coronary artery disease who were divided into cohorts treated with percutaneous coronary intervention and medication (n = 1274), CABG surgery and surgery (n = 1096), and medication alone (n = 516). Using multivariate analysis by Cox regression, they found that metabolic syndrome had no independent effect on survival regardless of the diabetic status of the patient.

Some have proposed clinicians should consider a weight-reduction strategy for the morbidly obese patient before surgery for CABG.[18] They believe preoperative fitness would be optimized and perioperative and postoperative complications minimized. Others disagree because a large percentage of morbidly obese patients have metabolic syndrome, which is associated with insulin resistance, dyslipidemia, and hypertension, along with proinflammatory and prothrombotic states.[19] They concluded that weight reduction alone is not enough to reduce the complications associated with CABG surgery in these patients.[19]

The STS considers diabetes to be an independent risk factor for death following CABG surgery.[20] Furnary and coworkers[20] have been studying the effect of strict glucose control in CABG surgery patients since 1987. They have demonstrated marked reductions in mortality and morbidity with their insulin infusion protocols and have raised the bar for glucose control in all patients undergoing cardiac surgery.

The implications for nursing practice are well established. Glucose levels should be monitored closely in postoperative cardiac surgery care. Insulin infusions with close glucose monitoring (at least hourly) and titration to maintain serum glucose levels between 90 to 150 mg/dL have been associated with improved patient outcomes.[20] There is an increase in the intensity of nursing care associated with the closer glucose monitoring, which has been documented as a significant dissatisfier for critical care nurses.[21]

Time to Extubation/Prolonged Ventilation

There have been inconsistent results by investigators who have studied ventilation times in obese patients following CABG surgery; however, several have reported longer ventilation times in moderately and extremely obese patients.[1,6] Ahn and colleagues[22] conducted a retrospective, continuous quality improvement audit of 200 randomly selected patients who underwent CABG surgery over a 2-year period. Their purpose was to determine if obesity affects postoperative intubation time when using a fast-track recovery strategy. Their definition for obesity was a BMI greater than 30.0 kg/m^2. Eighty-four (42%) of the patients met the obesity criteria and most were able to undergo the fast-track recovery process. Their time to extubation was prolonged and failure to be extubated was more common. Forty-six percent of patients in the obese group were able to be extubated in less than 2 hours compared with 63% in the non-obese group. At 6 hours, 85% of the obese patients were extubated compared with 98% of the non-obese patients. Ten of the obese patients required intubation longer than 12 hours.[22]

There are several factors that may contribute to the longer intubation time. Lung compliance in the obese patient is 35% lower than in the non-obese patient; this has been attributed to changes in lung or chest-wall compliance. Expiratory reserve volumes are lower related to the continuous weight gain.[23] Obese patients must therefore exert more diaphragmatic activity to overcome pulmonary elastance, which increases cardiac work load.[24] The respiratory muscles of an obese person must work twice as hard compared with a person who has normal BMI; therefore, these patients are at much greater risk for respiratory failure due to muscle fatigue.

A second issue is the higher incidence of obstructive sleep apnea (OSA) in this patient population. The patient should be screened for OSA preoperatively and plans made for postoperative ventilatory management using bilevel positive airway pressure (BiPAP) or continuous positive airway pressure (CPAP) once the patient has been extubated. If patients use BiPAP or CPAP at home, they are asked to bring their home equipment with them to the hospital. The nursing management of these patients following extubation to prevent the onset of acute respiratory failure indicates the patient be maintained in a sitting position at 30° to 45° to reduce abdominal pressure on the diaphragm and the work of breathing; this increases the patient's tidal volume.

Pain management should avoid excessive amounts of opioids, which can contribute to respiratory depression if the patient is opioid naïve.

When the patient is ready for transfer from the ICU, the handoff from the ICU nurse to the cardiac surgical floor nurse should include a detailed discussion regarding ventilatory status, use of BiPAP or CPAP, and pain management issues. The nursing staff should avoid the concomitant administration of pain medication with sleeping pills. Should the patient develop respiratory distress, this could lead to readmission to the ICU and reintubation. Of interest is a study examining causes of readmissions to a cardiac surgical ICU. The investigators conducted a retrospective chart review and found obesity (BMI > 30 kg/m^2) and respiratory failure were common causes of ICU readmission.[25] Readmission to the ICU was associated with a mortality rate of 30.8% and a longer ICU length of stay.[25]

Infections

Prabhakar and colleagues[1] and Jin and colleagues[7] reported a relative risk for deep sternal wound infections of 2.2% (95% CI, 2.01–2.45) in moderately obese patients and 3.15 (95% CI, 2.79–3.55) in extremely obese patients. Cardiopulmonary bypass times and use of internal mammary arteries were identical in both groups. Kuduvalli and coworkers[6] reported severely obese patients were more likely to have sternal wound infections (adjusted OR 2.10, $P = .038$) and 4.17 ($P = .001$) times more likely to have harvest site infections.

Others have demonstrated the increased incidence of sternal wound infections.[26] Researchers have been able to demonstrate a reduction in sternal wound infection rates with tighter glucose control.[20,26] Harrington and colleagues[26] suggested that in addition to glucose control, patients should be encouraged to lose weight before having CABG surgery. Performing a retrospective review of 4474 patients who underwent CABG surgery in Australia in five hospitals between August 1998 and May 2001, they learned that obesity was a major risk factor for surgical site infection (24.8%, RR 1.76, CI .095, χ^2 21.32, $P<.001$).

Activity Levels

Early postoperative mobilization of surgical patients is associated with fewer complications. The same is true for the CABG surgery patient. Nursing staff may be reluctant to assist the morbidly obese patient out of bed or promote early ambulation because of the perceived risk involved in needing to lift the patient. The morbidly obese patient is accustomed to carrying his or her weight. In many cases the nurse need only to instruct the patient on how to sit up in bed using the bed controls and subsequently move to the side of the bed to dangle without placing pressure on his or her arms, avoiding any pressure on the sternum. Positioning a walker or a wheelchair turned backward in front of the patient before standing assists in stabilizing the patient as he or she reaches the standing position.[23] The ambulation goals for this post-CABG surgery patient population are just as important as for other patients.

SUMMARY

There are many studies with significant numbers of obese patients investigating mortality and morbidity following CABG surgery. One of the major limitations applicable to all of the studies is the variation of definitions for obesity and severe obesity. Several conclusions can be drawn from these, however. The obese patient (BMI > 30 kg/m^2) does not have higher mortality rates than the non-obese CABG surgery patient. Pulmonary status and risk for respiratory failure are of concern in the nursing care of these patients. It is imperative that preoperative screening for OSA be performed with a structured plan for the management of these patients once extubated. The nurse-to-nurse handoff from the ICU to the post-cardiac surgery floor with effective communication about the use of BiPAP or CPAP is an important piece of the patient management across the continuum. Having this process in place can prevent unnecessary readmissions to the ICU and improve patient outcomes.

REFERENCES

1. Prabhakar G, Haaan CK, Peterson ED, et al. The risks of moderate and extreme obesity for coronary artery bypass grafting outcomes: a study from the Society of Thoracic Surgeons' Database. Ann Thorac Surg 2002;74:1125–31.
2. Lloyd-Jones D, Adams R, Carnethon M, et al. Heart disease and stroke statistics 2009 update. A report from the American Heart Association Statistics Committee and Stroke Statistics Subcommittee. Circulation 2008;108:191261 Available at: http://circ.ahajournals.org. Accessed December 18, 2008.
3. Birkmeyer NJO, Charlesworth DC, Hernandez F, et al. Obesity and risk of adverse outcomes associated with coronary artery bypass surgery. Circulation 1998;97: 1689–94.
4. Brandt M, Harder K, Walluscheck KP, et al. Severe obesity does not adversely affect perioperative mortality and morbidity in coronary artery bypass surgery. Eur J Cardiothorac Surg 2001;19:662–6.
5. Maurer MS, Luchsinger JA, Wellner R, et al. The effect of body mass index on complications from cardiac surgery in the oldest old. J Am Geriatr Soc 2002; 50(6):988–94.
6. Kuduvalli M, Grayson AD, Oo AY, et al. Risk of mortality in obese patients undergoing coronary artery bypass surgery. Eur J Cardiothorac Surg 2002;22:787–93.
7. Jin R, Grunkemeier GL, Furnary AP, et al. Is obesity a risk factor for mortality in coronary artery bypass surgery? (for the Providence Health System Cardiovascular Study Group). Circulation 2005;111:3359–65.
8. Lindhout AH, Wouters CW, Noyez L. Influence of obesity on in-hospital and early mortality and morbidity after myocardial revascularization. Eur J Cardiothorac Surg 2004;26:535–41.
9. Reeves BC, Ascione R, Chamberlain MH, et al. Effect of body mass index on early outcomes in patients undergoing coronary artery bypass surgery. J Am Coll Cardiol 2003;42:668–76.
10. Kim JK, Hammar N, Jakobsson K, et al. Obesity and the risk of early and late mortality after coronary artery bypass graft surgery. Am Heart J 2003;146: 555–60.
11. Engelman DT, Adams DH, Byrne JG, et al. Impact of body mass index and albumin on morbidity and mortality after cardiac surgery. J Thorac Cardiovasc Surg 1999;118:866–73.
12. Rockx MAJ, Fox SA, Stitt LW, et al. Is obesity a predictor of mortality, morbidity and readmission after cardiac surgery. Can J Surg 2004;47(1):34–8.
13. Gruberg L, Mercado N, Milo S, et al. Impact of body mass index on the outcome of patients with multivessel disease randomized to either coronary artery bypass grafting or stenting in the ARTS trial: the obesity paradox II? Am J Cardiol 2005; 95:439–44.
14. Habib RH, Zacharias A, Schwann TA. Effects if obesity and small body size on operative and long-term outcomes of coronary artery bypass surgery: a propensity-matched analysis. Ann Thorac Surg 2005;79:1976–86.

15. Isomaa B, Almgren P, Tuomi T, et al. Cardiovascular morbidity and mortality associated with the metabolic syndrome. Diabetes Care 2001;24(4):683–9.
16. Pan W, Hindler K, Lee V, et al. Obesity in diabetic patients undergoing coronary artery bypass graft surgery is associated with increased postoperative mortality. Anesthesiology 2006;104(6):441–7.
17. Shah B, Kumar N, Garg P, et al. Metabolic syndrome does not impact survival in patients treated for coronary artery disease. Coron Artery Dis 2008;19:71–7.
18. Elahi MM, Chetty GK, Sosnowski AW, et al. Morbid obesity increases perioperative morbidity in first-time CABG patients – should resources be redirected to weight reduction. Int J Cardiol 2005;105:98–9.
19. Turhan H, Yetkin E. Obesity-related increased perioperative morbidity in CABG patients: does metabolic syndrome affect perioperative outcomes? Int J Cardiol 2006;110:273–4.
20. Furnary AP, Gao G, Grunkemeier GL, et al. Continuous insulin infusion reduces mortality in patients with diabetes undergoing coronary artery bypass grafting. J Thorac Cardiovasc Surg 2003;125(5):1007–18.
21. Eigsti J, Henke K. Innovative solutions: development and implementation of a tight blood glucose management protocol. Dimens Crit Care Nurs 2006;25(2):62–5.
22. Ahn R, Parlow JL, Milne B. Does obesity affect time to extubation in "fast-track" CABG surgery? [abstract]. Can J Anaesth 2005;52(Suppl A28).
23. Davidson JE, Kruse MW, Cox DH, et al. Critical care of the morbidly obese. Crit Care Nurs Q 2002;26(2):105–16.
24. Charleboiss D, Wilmoth D. Critical care of patients with obesity. Crit Care Nurs 2004;24(4):19–27.
25. Chung DA, Sharples LD, Nashef SA. A case-control analysis of readmissions to the cardiac surgical intensive care unit. Eur J Cardiothorac Surg 2002;22:283–6.
26. Harrington G, Russo P, Spelman D, et al. Surgical-site infection rates and risk factor analysis in coronary artery bypass graft surgery. Infect Control Hosp Epidemiol 2004;25:472–6.

Trauma in Obese Patients: Implications for Nursing Practice

Sherry N. VanHoy, MSN, RN, ACNS-BC, CEN[a],*,
V. Tereceita Laidlow, MS, RN, CCRN[b]

KEYWORDS

- Trauma • Obesity • Clinical management
- Mechanism of injury • Initial resuscitation
- Pre-hospital care

Obesity has reached epidemic proportions internationally and the problem is no less significant in the United States. Once a problem primarily affecting adults, the obesity crisis has now become a national epidemic in adults and children of all ages. Obesity is defined as an excessive accumulation of body fat and is a chronic condition characterized by a slow, steady, progressive increase in body weight.[1] Obesity poses a major risk for many health conditions, including trauma. Consequently, every bodily system and anatomic structure can be affected by obesity. The economic impact on the health care system is so alarming that in 2001, the Surgeon General's Call to Action mentions grave medical consequences and economic burdens obesity inflects on society.[2]

Trauma is the fifth leading cause of death in the United States. When combined with obesity, the consequences can be grave. Recently, the impact of obesity on the outcomes of trauma patients has been the focus of several investigations. There have been several studies addressing the impact of obesity on trauma patients. These studies have explicated the impact of obesity on negative outcomes of trauma patients. Several studies have identified a relationship between obesity and injury pattern, increased complications in outcomes related to surgical procedures, and increase mortality and morbidity rates in obese trauma patients. However, the literature in nursing management in this patient population is virtually nonexistent and vague. The purpose of this article is to delineate the nursing implications of obesity in trauma patients and to provide guidelines for care of obese trauma patients.

According to the World Health Organization (WHO), there are more than 1 billion overweight adults; 300 million categorized as clinically obese.[3] The statistics are

[a] Department of Emergency Medicine, Sinai Hospital of Baltimore, 2401 W. Belvedere Avenue, Baltimore, MD 21215, USA
[b] Department of Nursing Administration, Sinai Hospital of Baltimore, 2401 W. Belvedere Avenue, Baltimore, MD 21215, USA
* Corresponding author.
E-mail address: svanhoy@lifebridgehealth.org (S.N. VanHoy).

Crit Care Nurs Clin N Am 21 (2009) 377–389
doi:10.1016/j.ccell.2009.07.004
0899-5885/09/$ – see front matter © 2009 Elsevier Inc. All rights reserved.

ccnursing.theclinics.com

equally astounding here in the United States. In the past 25 years, the obesity epidemic has affected more than 60 million adults. More than 20% of adults in the United States are obese revealing a 61% increase is since 1991. Alarmingly, this equates to 20% to 25% of the entire United States' population. The rate of obesity in children has increased even more dramatically. In the last decade, obesity in children has doubled for children aged 2 to 5 years and tripled for those aged 6 to 11 years.[4] In response to this trend, there has been growing research focusing on the impact of obesity on surgical interventions and medical diseases. Studies have shown that obesity and excess weight pose a major risk for many health conditions and debilitating diseases, including heart disease, type II diabetes, hypertension, stroke, respiratory problems, and some forms of cancers. Ironically, these are among the top ten health related issues in the United States, and include the top four causes of adult deaths in this country. Consequently, obesity is considered the leading cause of preventable death in the United States and accounts for more than 100,000 deaths annually, with an approximate cost of 1 billion dollars.[3]

Trauma ranks fifth as the cause of adult deaths in the United States and the leading cause of death in children and young adults aged 1 to 24 years. When trauma occurs in the overweight or obese population, it presents many challenges that negatively impact outcomes. The mortality rate for obese trauma patients is more than eight times that of victims whose weight is within normal parameters.[5] The statistics are so astonishing that many health care organizations, including the WHO and the Centers for Disease Control (CDC), are calling for a healthier America by 2010 and 2020.[3,4]

As prevalence of obesity in the trauma population increases, nurses are confronted with the challenges and complexities associated with effective management of these patients. Among the principal challenges for nurses and providers are obtaining a comprehensive assessment, meeting patients' physiologic requirements, providing timely and effective intervention, and maintaining vigilance in ongoing evaluation and discharge. Paramount to providing optimal nursing care is recognition for early planning and preparation, if possible before arrival, and maintained throughout the continuum of care. It is essential that nurses caring for obese trauma patients have an understanding of their anatomic, physical, and psychological needs, and any special equipment or requirements for the patients. Unfortunately, many nurses and institutions are ill-equipped to provide specialized care required for this population of patients.

DEFINITION AND CLASSIFICATIONS OF OBESITY IN ADULT/PEDIATRIC POPULATIONS

Obesity is generally defined as having an abnormally increased proportion of adipose tissue or body fat in relation to muscle mass.[6] The most popular method to determine obesity is calculating the body mass index (BMI) (Appendix).[7] BMI is a simple mathematical calculation in which the weight in kilograms is divided by the height in meters square (weight [kg]/height [m2]). In children and teens, BMI is calculated using a BMI-for-age that considers the normal difference in body fat between boys and girls as they mature. Calculations for BMI are categorized from under weight to obese (**Table 1**). Obesity increases the risk of developing adverse health conditions that can cause further complications when the individual suffers from injury.[8]

MECHANISM OF INJURY AND BIOMECHANICS

Injury results when the body is exposed to an excessive form of energy, such as kinetic (crash, fall, bullet), chemical, thermal, electrical or radiation, or from a lack of essential agents, such as oxygen or heat (drowning and frostbite). Mechanics of injury are related to the type of injury force and subsequent tissue response. The degree of injury

Table 1	
Body mass index classification of obesity	
BMI	**Weight Status**
Below 18.5	Under weight
18.5–24.9	Normal
25.5–29.9	Over weight
30.0 and above	Obese

varies according to the presence of accompanying factors, such as severity of injury, age, gender, geography, alcohol and obesity. These factors increase the incidence of morbidity and mortality after a trauma. Trauma centers across the country can expect an increase in admissions of obese injured patients. A thorough understanding of mechanism of injury can help explain the type of injury, predict outcome, and identify common combinations of injuries. Acquiring such knowledge can improve nursing management and care of the obese trauma patient.

Blunt trauma can be categorized as any type of injury to the body that is caused by direct impact, such as physical attacks, falls, and motor-vehicle collisions. Motor-vehicle collisions continue to be the leading cause of injury-related death in the United States and accounted for more than 45,500 deaths in 2005.[8] Injury patterns and severity of injury ultimately depend on factors, such as speed, velocity changes, seat belt usage, airbag deployment, and type of collision.[9] Recent literature reveals the differences of injuries from motor-vehicle collisions in obese patients from nonobese patients.

Between 2000 and 2005, the Crash Injury Research and Engineering Network study reviewed crash statistics of 1615 individuals more than 16 years of age. The study investigated what influence obesity would have on patients' outcomes from motor-vehicle collisions. During their research, they found a pattern of higher incidence of thoracic, pelvic, and lower extremity injuries, and a lower incidence of head injuries.[10] Similar injury patterns from motor-vehicle crashes were found in a retrospective report by Byrnes and colleagues.[11] During their study, 1179 trauma patients more than 18 years of age were reviewed and they found an increase of extremity and pelvic fractures and pulmonary injuries in obese patients or who had a BMI greater than or equal to 35. Even though pulmonary injuries were more prevalent in the obese population, the occurrence of pneumothorax and intra-abdominal injuries were lower.[12] Increased thoracic body mass or waist circumference typically seen in obese individuals may explain these patterns. This enlargement could provide some increased protection to intra-abdominal vital organs, however obese individuals will also have increased body fat that will increase the force in which the body contacts in a collision. The end result is usually dashboard and steering wheel injuries.[13] These injuries support the above findings of increased pelvic and lower extremity injuries. In contrast, a study done by Brown and colleagues,[14] involving 690 patients, found less skull fractures in the obese population. However, traumatic brain injury remains the leading cause of death. They hypothesized that higher mortality was caused by other factors, such as age and hypotension on arrival to the hospital, and not the obese state. Other blunt trauma injuries include falls resulting in sprains, strains, and dislocations.[15] Such musculoskeletal injuries are most likely caused by decreased mobility and overexertion. Where children are concerned, those who are overweight are at an increase for ankle injuries.[16]

Regardless of the patterns of injury, mortality from blunt trauma was found to be higher (42%) among obese individuals than normal-weight persons (5%). The increase in mortality is directly related to complications resulting from the trauma.[10]

PREHOSPITALIZATION AND INITIAL RESUSCITATION

The ultimate goal of the prehospital phase is to stabilize and transport trauma patients to an appropriate level trauma facility. The emergency medical service (EMS) is central to the coordination of an effective and efficient process. Specially trained paramedics must communicate with a centralized communication center and the trauma facility physician or nursing staff to assist with planning the appropriate mode of transport for patients. Obese trauma patients are especially at risk during this phase when time is critical. Conditions at the scene may necessitate a call for additional personnel, such as firefighters, to help with extrication, or police officials to direct traffic to prevent further injuries. Often, additional equipment, such as oversized or dual backboards, may be required to accommodate morbidly obese patients. Cervical collars are not large enough or will not always fit properly to maintain cervical spine stabilization, resulting in the use of other options available at the time. Sandbags, blanket rolls, and tape are alternate resources that can be used for neck stabilization until possible cervical injuries can be eliminated.[5] Obese patients have an increased risk of lower extremity fractures therefore stabilizing fractures will be challenging.[15] Most splints will not fit obese patients, so again, tape or elastic bandages will be required for stabilization. Many ambulances have added stretchers that can accommodate 750 lbs; however getting them on the stretcher requires extra manpower, unique stabilization techniques, and additional time. These complications can result in increased extrication and transport times, which can delay life-saving treatment in severely injured patients. Some communities have interdisciplinary teams of EMS, nurses, and physicians called "go teams" to assist in the care and transportation en route. More recently, flight trauma nursing is a growing specialty in many states but there are strict weight considerations for air transport. Care of obese trauma patients necessitates a well-orchestrated, preplanned approach that should include a complete prehospital report, knowledge of the equipment needed, and possible alteration in standards of care to provide positive outcomes. Prehospital reports provide valuable information for the facility health care team, such as number of backboards required for transportation, nonfitting cervical collar, extrication challenges, or the need for extra crew. It is also critical to have medical and surgical history regarding the patient, including comorbidities, which allows the emergency medical personnel to anticipate complications and provide appropriate interventions en route to the trauma center.

A vital part of the prehospital process is obtaining a comprehensive history of patients. This process is often very difficult because trauma patients may or maybe not be able to verbalize personal or health care information. Having a list of information, such as legal next of kin and their contact information, diseases, medications, and allergies, are helpful in times of emergencies, such as trauma. In the past 5 years, many states are recommending that their residents carry an In Case of Emergency card. The card offers a comprehensive method for communicating essential personal information to health care providers in the event you are incapacitated. In the case of obese patients, information about past medical history regarding bariatric surgeries is equally important data. In the initial evaluation of obese trauma patients, a careful history of the events leading up to the injury must be obtained. A quick survey of the scene and interrogation of observers and patients may reveal essential information. Aspects of the scene and surrounding damages provide clues to potential injuries and aid in diagnosis.

ASSESSMENT AND CLINICAL MANAGEMENT

The Advance Trauma Life Support guidelines for initial assessment provide a standardized approach for care of trauma patients. Standardization of language and care process enhances communication with all members of the emergency team in the field and at the trauma and command centers. Trauma care involves the use of basic assessment priorities: airway, breathing, and circulation (ABC).[17]

Airway

Maintaining airway patency is the foundation of emergency resuscitation. Patients who are morbidly obese are at risk for compromised airway because excess adipose tissue increases the work of breathing when the patient is in a supine position. Additionally, these patients have an increase risk for aspiration caused by gastroesophageal reflux and increased abdominal pressure.[18] When emergency airway control is needed, obese patients present an intubation challenge for health care providers and anesthesia. Many of these difficult airways result in the inability to acquire successful intubation or unintended esophageal intubation. Excess neck tissue may mask crucial anatomic landmarks required for surgical airways, such as tracheotomy or surgical cricothyrotomy, should one be required. In addition, obese patients are at risk for complications, such as pneumothoraces, aspiration, atelectasis, or arrhythmias.[19] Trauma patients may require supplemental high-oxygen delivery by way of face mask; however obtaining a proper fit may be difficult because of excess facial tissue. Some obese patients are prone to sleep apnea and can obstruct their airway when lying flat, however this position is a standard of care for spinal immobilization of trauma patients. Obese patients have reduced lung volumes and compliance resulting in ventilation/perfusion mismatch.[20] Nurses and other members of the health care team need to be mindful of these issues and be prepared to deliver oxygen through an alternative route, such as bivalve positive airway pressure.[18]

Breathing

Diagnosing blunt traumatic injuries of the chest can be difficult because auscultation and percussion is not feasible because of the cushion effect from subcutaneous tissue. An alternative assessment option is palpation of the chest wall for crepitus from subcutaneous air. Additionally, oxygenation and increases in carbon dioxide retention is probable. Obese patients tend to have lower oxygen saturation on high oxygen delivery. For example, saturation may be as low as 88% to 92% on 6 L/minute by face mask. Monitoring techniques, such as arterial blood gases or placement of an arterial catheter, is recommended to ensure adequate oxygenation.

Circulation

Obesity has significant impact on the cardiovascular system. These patients have greater perfusion needs because of an increase in adipose tissue resulting in an already amplified stoke volume, cardiac output, and an increase left ventricular workload leading to left ventricular dilation and hypertrophy. The end result is an increase in hypoxia and hypercapnia.[18] Although fluid resuscitation is one of the gold standards of trauma care, in obese patients, fluid resuscitation should be managed with caution.[6]

Disability

Beginning with arrival to the emergency department, challenges in providing care and resuscitation of obese trauma patients can be difficult. Proper apparatus for removal of patients from the ambulance to the trauma bay may require additional equipment for safe transfer. Immediately following attention to ABC, emergency resuscitation providers should note the patients' neurologic status. Baseline neurologic assessment must include level of consciousness and pupillary size and reaction. Change in mental status is an early indication of traumatic head injury. Studies have shown obese trauma patients have a lower incidence of head injuries, but rationale was not noted.[10] External evidence of trauma and mechanism of injury should alert the nurses and other members of the health care team of the possibility of internal injuries. These signs may be easily overlooked in any trauma especially when obvious hemorrhage and wounds are visible. This problem is even more prevalent in obese patients, because some body areas do not lend themselves to physical examination because of extra adipose tissue. Ryb and Dischinger[10] studied the injury severity and outcome of 1615 over-weight and obese patients after vehicular trauma. They found that obese trauma patients have a lower incidence of abdominal injury because of the cushioning effects of fat around the abdominal area, but a higher incidence of thoracic and lower extremity injuries. While the reason for the higher incidence of thoracic and lower extremity injuries in obese trauma patients was not noted, the author hypothesized that less adipose tissue, inactivity, and poor nutrition may have weakened large bony structures of the chest and legs.

TRAUMA RESUSCITATION

A coordinated, collaborative, and unified approach to trauma care during the resuscitative phase is imperative in all cases, but even more critical in the obese trauma. Most facilities are well equipped to meet the needs of most traumas with normal to overweight BMI score. However, obese patients with a BMI greater than 30 require special equipment including: access to the trauma area; location of the trauma area to the operating room; size and location of the elevators; size and weight capacity of diagnostic apparatus, such as CT scanners; beds and stretchers; and blood pressure cuff, to name a few. Advance preparation for immediate availability of equipment, supplies, and personnel that patients might need for survival and prompt care is essential. As a result, communication with the prehospital team is crucial to adequately prepare for the arrival of patients, as every second lost decreases the patients' chance of survival. Notification before arrival allows the facility to mobilize and adequately prepare the trauma team. On arrival to the trauma or emergency care facility, orderly transition from field to hospital trauma team is crucial.

During patient assessment, the resuscitation team plays a vital role in the evaluation and stabilization of obese trauma patients upon admission. There are many challenges to the care of obese trauma patients. Equipment limitations, pain management requirements, difficulty positioning obese patients, and an increase in complexity in performing procedures often complicate therapeutic and diagnostic interventions. With trauma patients, assessment and plan of care necessitate a team approach. The team consists of surgeons, emergency physicians, emergency nurses, respiratory therapist, and other support staff. The initial focus is to perform a primary and secondary survey of patients to promptly identify life-threatening injuries. Given the size of obese patients, additional staff may be necessary to turn, position, and transport patients during this phase. It is crucial to have enough help to perform these tasks safely to prevent injury to patients and members of the trauma team. The primary assessment commences with an initial survey of ABC as was performed during the prehospital phase. The nursing team needs to maintain the continuum of assessment by repeating the primary survey as done before arrival. The goal of continuous assessment of primary functions is to assist the team in rapidly identifying changes in airway, breathing, and circulation.[21]

Secondary assessment is the hallmark of the hospital resuscitation phase. During the secondary assessment, special attention is given to bodily injuries using a systematic approach. In addition, monitoring and assessing pulmonary function and oxygenation is important. Pulse oximetry is not always accurate because of increased adipose tissue creating a barrier for the penetration of the light sensor.[6] Nursing should use alternate placement areas of the body, such as the bridge of the nose or earlobe, to obtain a measurement. As discussed earlier, auscultation of breath sounds will be difficult because of increases in body fat. An attempt to sit patients upright will require increased nursing support. Similar to listening to breath sounds, heart sounds will also prove difficult to hear. Nurses can sit patients upright to bring the heart closer to the chest wall to assess for murmurs or other adventitious sounds. While assessing cardiovascular function, jugular vein distention can predict heart failure and evidence of trauma-related lung or chest injury. For example, routine measurement of vital signs can be challenging in obese patients. Regular or large blood pressure cuffs may not fit obese patients. To obtain an accurate measurement, the cuff should be greater than or equal to 40% of the patients' arm circumference.[6] Alternate methods, such as thigh cuffs, should be used; however, fit and placement may lead to inaccurate results. Equally important to hemodynamic monitoring is the ability to assess circulation. Obese individuals may have increased extremity swelling caused by immobility and venous stasis.[6] Peripheral pulse assessment can be difficult to attain with increases in body tissue, so nursing should anticipate the need for Doppler assessment to aid in their cardiovascular assessment. Other diagnostic equipment may be used in identifying internal injuries, such as noninvasive procedures.

When circulation is compromised, fluid resuscitation is the standard of care. Again, it is important to remember that obese patients have a decrease ability to withstand shock.[6] Traditionally, large bore intravenous (IV) access is necessary for volume resuscitation in trauma. However, in obese patients obtaining IV, access may be impossible because of large amounts of subcutaneous tissue. Other options may be needed, such as central venous catheters, interosseous, or as a last resort, internal venous cutdown.

Some radiographic studies are not feasible in the obese population. Portable chest X ray is feasible in obese patients and easier if taken with the head of bed elevated at 10 to 15 degrees. Unfortunately, because of excess tissue, obtaining clear images is challenging. CT may be the best method to identify lung and chest injuries.[18] It is important to know the weight limitation of the CT scanner of your facility. Unless a specialized bariatric surgery center, most CT scanners are limited to approximately 350 pounds. Often, obese patients may require X rays of the extremities. However, additional personnel may be required to support the extremity during radiological studies. To illuminate abdominal injuries, the Focused Assessment with Sonography for Trauma (FAST) examination is a bedside ultrasound imaging tool is used with increasing prevalence with notable success for diagnosing internal injuries. In obese patients, the FAST examination is useless because of visceral and subcutaneous tissue.[18] If internal bleeding is suspected, diagnostic peritoneal lavage is contraindicated because of the inability to identify appropriate landmarks and inappropriate size of the catheter.

Incidence of gastroesophageal disease, such as reflux, hiatal hernia, and increased abdominal pressure, in obese patients perpetuate the risk of aspiration. Placement of tubes to decompress the abdomen, such as nasogastric/orogastric tubes, may be warranted. In addition, it is important to monitor urine output in trauma patients to evaluate renal function. Foley catheter placement are often challenging in obese patients because of the need for additional persons to assist with displacement of skin folds to aid in visualization.

Some trauma patients may need immediate surgical intervention. Like the emergency department, additional personnel may be required to assist with transport and transfer of obese patients. Operating room beds may not be adequate to accommodate obese patients, therefore larger size beds may be necessary. Depending on the surgical procedure, proper positioning may be required to lessen the potential for skin breakdown and nerve damage.[5] Positioning of extremities may need extra, such as stirrups and arm boards, which will require sheets or other fastening devices leading to excessive pressure on the skin. As a result, frequent assessment of the skin is important during the procedure. Of greater concern is the choice of anesthetics for morbidly obese patients. Local or regional anesthesia may be given, but locating landmarks may prove challenging. Additionally, spinal and epidural anesthesia may not be possible because of incorrect length of the spinal needle. If percutaneous administration of pain medication is not possible postoperatively, adequate pain control may be difficult as medication may not be easily absorbed by other routes except intravenously. As discussed previously, landmarks for intravenous placement are not always visible or palpable.

INTRAHOSPITAL PHASE

Postoperative care of patients begins during the intraoperative phase. The goal of intraoperative care is to monitor vital signs, pain control, and assess for complications, such as hemorrhage. When critically injured obese patients are admitted to the unit, the potential complications are prevalent. The literature supports an increase in mortality of 10% to 20% in obese patients versus nonobese patients.[10,11,20,22] Obese patients have higher incidence of multiorgan failures and other complications.[22,23] Common complications include:

Multiple system organ failure
Pneumonia
Sepsis
Acute respiratory distress syndrome
Renal failure
Myocardial infraction
Deep vein thrombosis (DVT)
Pulmonary embolism (PE)

Mechanical ventilation is often necessary in critically ill obese trauma patients to maintain adequate ventilation and perfusion. Trauma patients with thoracic injuries are particularly prone to pulmonary shunting, dead space ventilation, and reduced tidal volume.[13] Ventilator settings for obese patients are usually higher than for nonobese patients including, increase rate, tidal volume, and the addition of positive end expiratory pressure. Obese patients produce copious amounts of respiratory secretion rendering them at risk for aspiration. Therefore, frequent suctioning, oral care, and elevation of the head of the bed may help to prevent aspiration and ventilator associated pneumonia. Specialty beds should be acquired when patients are admitted because it helps to loosen pulmonary secretions, aids in ventilation, and prevents skin breakdown. Placement of patients within the first 24 hours is important to be effective.[6] Even with proper ventilation management, literature supports an increased amount of ventilator days and difficulty with extubation compared with non-obese patients.[23]

Medication management is an essential element of care for critically ill patients. Excessive adipose tissue alters absorption and distribution of medication causing subtherapeutic or toxic levels. It is important to monitor the patients' response to medication to determine effectiveness. Frequent reassessment of pain levels by the nursing staff is necessary for proper pain management. Adequate pain control is necessary to promote wellness. To optimize pharmacologic effects, a team approach is helpful and should include nurses, pharmacists, and physicians.

In the event of cardiac arrest, cardiopulmonary resuscitation (CPR) needs to be initiated. However, effectiveness of CPR may be hindered because of excess adipose tissue. Repositioning in a reverse Trendelenburg may help to decrease intra-abdominal pressure on the diaphragm and will provide more effective compressions.

A major complication of inactive obese patients is DVT. Morbidly obese patients have increase risk for DVT caused by inactivity, hypercoagulopathy, and the traumatic injury. Prophylactic treatment for DVT includes early ambulation and sequential compressive devices. Many of these compression devices may not fit properly on obese patients with large lower extremities, therefore these individuals should be treated with subcutaneous, or on rare occasions, intravenous doses of unfractionated or low-molecular weight heparin. The benefit of coagulation treatment must be weighed against the risk. If patients have a high risk for PE then insertion of a filter in the inferior vena cava is strongly recommended. Patients at risk for PE include those with venous stasis, BMI greater than 60, obstructive sleep apnea, truncal obesity, hypoventilation, and other conditions in which there are increased risk for clotting.

Protocol for the management of obese patients should include wound and aggressive skin care including frequent inspection. Obese patients have excess fat causing increase in body temperature and perspiration. The excess moisture is ideal for creating conditions conducive to irritation, skin breakdown, and bacteria. They are therefore prone to dermatitis, delayed wound healing, and ulceration. The most likely areas are neck, under breast, abdomen, and perineal areas. To minimize these problem areas, soft gauze can be placed between skin folds to prevent irritation. Powder is not recommended because it may contain abrasive particles and act as a medium for bacterial growth. Tubes and lines need to be assessed ensuring they are not embedded in skin folds which can lead to pressure ulcers. In addition, obese patients should be turned and repositioned every 2 hours to prevent skin breakdown. Urine and fecal incontinence are common and is attributed to increase abdominal pressure on the bladder.[24] Skin should be kept clean and dry at all times. Morbidly obese patients have difficulties with self care and nursing should be comfortable with assisting patients.

Obese trauma patients may have surgical and traumatic wounds. Patients who have open wounds may need dressing changes more frequently with complete wound assessment, including full description of wound, drainage, color, and odor if any. Abdominal binders may provide some support to dressings and offer pain relief. Morbidly obese patients have a greater tendency of wound dehiscence and infection caused by poor vascularity of the adipose tissue.[6]

Obese trauma patients are at risk for nutritional difficulties and undernourishment because of malabsorption and restrictive issues. Traumatic insults to obese patients may result in an increase of insulin production in combination with increase insulin resistance causing an increase in insulin needs. Severe elevation in glucose in obese patients can result in significant diuresis, diabetic ketoacidosis and diabetic coma.[24]

Therefore, judicious glucose monitoring and attention to insulin administration are essential parts of nursing care of obese trauma patients. Research shows that as many as 30% of obese patients already have some form of eating disorder and when combined with trauma, the problem is exacerbated. During stressful situations metabolic needs of patients are met by hypermetabolism and increase protein catabolism. Therefore, obese patients are susceptible to increased depletion of nutrients and large amounts of weight loss. They may lose fat and lean muscle mass resulting in protein malnutrition. Lean body mass may be in the form of muscle tissue, which can result in delays in ventilator weaning, rehabilitation, and early mobility. A high carbohydrate diet is important to decrease protein catabolism. Experts recommend a complete nutritional analysis of obese trauma patients. Enteral tube feeding or parenteral nutrition is needed in obese trauma patients who are unable to consume an oral diet. Estimating nutritional requirements may be a challenge because of the lack of consistency in the literature regarding nutritional needs of obese trauma patients. Practically, caloric needs may be determined by the patients' energy expenditure. Enteral nutrition should be based on 20 to 30 kcal/kg/day.[21]

PSYCHOSOCIAL

Many obese individuals live with massive psychological burden and suffering.[25] There are many societal attitudes toward the obese population and nurses need to be keenly aware of their own feelings regarding obesity. Although unintentional, health care providers identify obese patients with increased workload and unsuccessful treatment goals.[25] Nurses and health care providers need to be aware of obese patients' emotional needs and evaluate for signs of psychological distress, such as depression, shame, and low self-esteem. Open communication is essential between patients and their caregivers to identify needs for psychosocial support. Chaplain, social services, and psychiatric consultations should be anticipated. Obese patients may require additional assistance with care, therefore the patients' privacy and respect need to be maintained to promote positive self-image. Family and friends should be encouraged to participate in phases of care to provide emotional support and well being.

Equally important is to establish institutional guidelines and educational programs to provide optimal care of obese patients. In addition, nursing education needs to involve proper lifting techniques and application of available equipment to prevent provider and patient injury.

EVALUATION AND DISCHARGE PLANNING

Obese patients require additional resources to attain similar outcomes as nonobese trauma patients. Although obesity is not recognized as a comorbidity, its impact on the patients' health poses associated risk factors consistent with mortality after trauma. Continuity of care from admission through discharge is essential for trauma patients. The importance of rehabilitation is equally important to the quality of life patients can resume after discharge. Part of the recovery plan is to obtain the necessary consultations early to assist patients with therapies needed to begin their recuperation and prepare them for the best possible outcome. Most trauma patients require numerous referrals while hospitalized to provide assistance toward wellness. Obese patients pose challenges for the rehabilitation process because of the need for larger equipment. Most trauma centers include physical/occupational therapy programs.[11] Early ambulation should be promoted as early as possible to advance wound healing and prevent the occurrence of DVT. To make mobility less challenging, consider a larger or private room with plenty of space to move. Other tools include wide wheelchairs, walkers, and large chairs, such as recliners, to fit their needs. Members of the therapy team can provide medical equipment for their discharge needs. Collaboration with a wound care nurse can prevent and treat skin breakdown. Dieticians, social services, and a clinical nurse specialist should also be consulted, if available, to meet the needs of this special population.

Case managers will need to be consulted to determine the needs of patients before discharge to home or an extended care facility. They need to investigate numerous resources including payer sources, equipment needs, and family support. If they are unable to ambulate or injuries have left them confined, stairs and other barriers in the home need to be identified. For long-term facilities, there may be difficulty in finding an appropriate facility that can offer the needed equipment for obese patients. Discharge planning begins as soon as possible to prevent increased length of stays in the hospital. Nurses have the opportunity to provide education regarding the effects of obesity and promote wellness in the community.

SUMMARY

Complications from trauma are exaggerated in the obese population. These patients have numerous comorbidities that negatively affect outcomes after trauma. Literature supports that changes in the practice guidelines that include considerations of obese patients can decrease length of stay, mortality, and morbidity. As obesity and bariatric programs become more prevalent, nurses will need to remain current in unique practice methods, including available products, equipment, and evidence-based recommendations. While these patients present a level of anxiety in nurses, proper education involving patient care and nurse safety can be an effective method of support.

Further research is needed to examine the impact of recommended practice guidelines on the outcome of obese trauma patients. In addition, more studies are needed to investigate the impact of implementation of recommended guidelines on attitudes of nurses, safety, and quality of care.

REFERENCES

1. Gallagher SM. Restructuring the therapeutic environment to promote care and safety for the obese patient. J Wound Ostomy Continence Nurs 1999;25:292–7.
2. American Obesity Association. Costs of obesity. Available at: http://obesity1. tempdomainname.com/treatment/cost.shtml. Accessed February 16, 2009.
3. World Health Organization. Obesity and overweight. Available at: http://www.who. int/dietphysicalactivity/publications/facts/obesity/en/. Accessed March 17, 2009.
4. Centers for Disease Control and Prevention. Obesity and overweight: introduction. Available at: http://www.cdc.gov/NCCDPHP/DNPA/obesity/. Accessed March 20, 2009.
5. Bushard S. Trauma in patients who are morbidly obese. AORN J 2002;76(4): 585–9.
6. Garrett K, Lauer K, Christopher B. The effects of obesity on the cardiopulmonary system: implications for critical care nursing. Prog Cardiovasc Nurs 2004 (Fall); 19(4):155–61.
7. National Heart, Lung and Blood Institute. BMI body mass index table. Available at: http://www.nhlbi.nih.gov/guidelines/obesity/bmi_tbl.pdf. Accessed March 20, 2009.

8. Centers for Disease Control and Prevention. Motor vehicle-related death rates–United States, 1999–2005. Available at: http://www.cdc.gov/ncip/osp/charts.htm. Accessed March 27, 2009.

9. Zhu S, Layde PM, Guse CE, et al. Obesity and risk for death due to motor vehicle crashes. Am J Public Health 2006;96(4):734–9.

10. Ryb GE, Dischinger PC. Injury severity and outcome of overweight and obese patients after vehicular trauma: a crash injury research and engineering network (CIREN) study. J Trauma 2008;64(2):406–11.

11. Byrnes MC, McDaniel MD, Moore MB, et al. The effect of obesity on outcomes among injured patients. J Trauma 2005;58:232–7.

12. Blackwell L, Clayton J, Marr AB, et al. Impact of obesity on associated injury and outcome in a blunt chest trauma cohort. [abstracts of papers to be presented at the Eighteenth Annual Scientific Meeting of the Eastern Association for the Surgery of Trauma. January 11-15, 2005 Ft. Lauderdale, (FL). J Trauma 2004; 57(6):1386.

13. Reiff DA, Hipp G, McGwin G Jr, et al. Body mass index affects the need for and the duration of mechanical ventilation. J Trauma 2007;62(6):1432–5.

14. Brown CV, Rhee P, Neville AL, et al. Obesity and traumatic brain injury. J Trauma 2006;61:572–6.

15. Matter KC, Sinclair SA, Hostetler SG, et al. A comparison of the characteristics of injuries between obese and non-obese inpatients. Obesity 2007;15:2384–90.

16. Zonfrillo MR, Seiden JA, House EM, et al. The association of overweight and ankle injuries in children. Ambul Pediatr 2008;8(1):66–9.

17. American College of Surgeons. Advanced trauma life support for doctors. 7th edition. Chicago: American College of Surgeons; 2004. p. 11–40.

18. Zigler MK. Obesity and the trauma patient: challenges and guidelines for care. J Trauma Nurs 2006;13(1):22–7.

19. Sifri ZC, Kim H, Lavery R, et al. The impact of obesity on the outcome of emergency intubation in trauma patients. J Trauma 2008;65:396–400.

20. Neville AL, Brown CV, Weng BS, et al. Obesity is an independent risk factor of mortality in severely injured blunt trauma patients. Arch Surg 2004;139:983–7.

21. Szczensiak SL. Trauma in the bariatric patient. In: McQuillan KA, Makic MF, Whalen E, editors. Trauma nursing: from resuscitation through rehabilitation. St. Louis (MO): Saunders/Elsevier; 2009. p. 850.

22. Brown CV, Neville AL, Rhee P, et al. The impact of obesity on the outcomes of 1153 critically injured blunt trauma patients. J Trauma 2005;59:1048–51.

23. Brown CV, Velmahos GC. The consequences of obesity on trauma, emergency surgery, and surgical critical care. World J Emerg Surg 2006;1(27):1–5.

24. Barth MM, Jenson CE. Postoperative nursing care of gastric bypass patients. Am J Crit Care 2006;15(4):378–87.

25. Hurst S, Blanco K, Boyle D, et al. Bariatric implications of critical care nursing. Dimens Crit Care Nurs 2004;23(2):76–83.

APPENDIX: BODY MASS INDEX TABLE

	Normal						Overweight					Obese										Extreme Obesity															
BMI	19	20	21	22	23	24	25	26	27	28	29	30	31	32	33	34	35	36	37	38	39	40	41	42	43	44	45	46	47	48	49	50	51	52	53	54
Height (inches)																Body Weight (Pounds)																				
58	91	96	100	105	110	115	119	124	129	134	138	143	148	153	158	162	167	172	177	181	186	191	196	201	205	210	215	220	224	229	234	239	244	248	253	258
59	94	99	104	109	114	119	124	128	133	138	143	148	153	158	163	168	173	178	183	18	193	198	203	208	212	217	222	227	232	237	242	247	252	257	262	267
60	97	102	107	112	118	123	128	133	138	143	148	153	158	163	168	174	179	184	189	194	199	204	209	215	220	225	230	235	240	245	250	255	261	266	271	276
61	100	106	111	116	122	127	132	137	143	148	153	158	164	169	174	180	185	190	195	201	206	211	217	222	227	232	238	243	248	254	259	264	269	275	280	285
62	104	109	115	120	126	131	136	142	147	153	158	164	169	175	180	186	191	196	202	07	213	218	224	229	235	240	246	251	256	262	267	273	278	284	289	295
63	107	113	118	124	130	135	141	146	152	158	163	169	175	180	186	191	197	203	208	214	220	225	231	237	242	248	254	259	265	270	278	282	287	293	299	304
64	110	116	122	128	134	140	145	151	157	163	169	174	180	186	192	197	204	209	215	221	227	232	238	244	250	256	262	267	273	279	285	291	296	302	308	314
65	114	120	126	132	138	144	150	156	162	168	174	180	186	192	198	204	210	216	222	228	234	240	246	252	258	264	270	276	282	28	294	300	306	312	318	324
66	118	124	130	136	142	148	155	161	167	173	179	186	192	198	204	210	216	223	229	235	241	247	253	260	266	272	278	284	291	297	303	309	315	322	328	334
67	121	127	134	140	146	153	159	166	172	178	185	191	198	204	211	217	223	230	236	242	249	255	261	268	274	280	287	293	299	306	312	319	325	331	338	344
68	125	131	138	144	151	158	164	171	177	184	190	197	203	210	216	223	230	236	243	249	256	262	269	276	282	289	295	302	30	315	322	328	335	341	348	354
69	128	135	142	149	155	162	169	176	182	189	196	203	209	216	223	230	236	243	250	257	263	270	277	284	291	297	304	311	318	324	331	338	345	351	358	365
70	132	139	146	153	160	167	174	181	188	195	202	29	216	222	229	236	243	250	257	264	271	278	285	292	299	306	313	320	327	334	341	348	355	362	369	376
71	136	143	150	157	165	172	179	186	193	200	208	215	222	229	235	242	250	257	265	272	279	287	294	302	309	316	324	331	338	346	353	361	368	375	383	390
72	140	147	154	162	169	177	184	191	199	206	213	221	228	235	242	250	258	265	272	279	287	294	302	309	316	324	331	338	346	353	361	368	375	383	390	397
73	144	151	159	166	174	182	189	197	204	212	219	227	235	242	250	257	265	272	280	28	295	302	310	318	325	333	340	348	355	363	371	378	386	393	401	408
74	148	155	63	171	179	186	194	202	210	218	225	233	241	249	256	264	272	280	287	295	303	311	319	326	334	342	350	358	365	373	381	389	396	404	412	420
75	152	160	168	176	184	192	200	208	216	224	232	240	248	256	264	272	279	287	295	303	311	319	327	335	343	351	359	367	375	383	391	399	407	415	423	431
76	156	164	172	180	189	197	205	213	221	230	238	246	254	263	271	279	287	295	304	312	320	328	336	344	353	361	369	377	385	394	402	410	418	426	435	443

Obesity-related Risks and Prevention Strategies for Critically Ill Adults

Margaret McAtee, MN, RN[a],*, Rebecca J. Personett, PhD[b]

KEYWORDS

- Bariatric • Body fat • Critically ill adults • Obesity
- Patient risks • Prevention

In America today, more than one third of adults are obese. These individuals have increased risk for a multitude of health disorders including diabetes, coronary artery disease, dyslipidemia, stroke, hypertension, gallbladder disease, certain cancers, osteoarthritis, sleep apnea and other respiratory disorders.[1] As the prevalence of obesity in the population has increased there has also been an increasing trend in hospitalized patients who are obese and morbidly obese. Their admission to critical care units exposes obese patients to an environment that may be unsuited to their special needs. Critical care nurses must have additional knowledge and skills to identify health risks to obese patients and implement interventions to prevent untoward problems. Critical care nurses are also at risk when taking care of obese patients. In this article, the authors introduce the scope of the problem, identify the underlying pathophysiology of obese patients that make them unique, identify obesity-related risks to the patient, suggest strategies to promote safe passage of the obese adult, and identify risks to critical care nursing staff and prevention strategies staff may use to avoid injury to themselves and to the hospitalized obese and morbidly obese patients.

Being overweight refers to an excess of weight, whereas obesity is described as having an excess of body fat.[2] Factors that can contribute to being overweight include weight from muscle, bone, fat, or body water; therefore, it is possible to be overweight without being obese. The most common screening tool used as a guideline to compare weight to risks is the body mass index (BMI). This index is a measure of weight in kilograms adjusted for height but does not measure actual body fat percentage, nor is it gender specific. The BMI is not meant to be diagnostic, but as a monitor to identify trends. The calculation is performed by dividing the weight by

[a] Education Department, Baylor All Saints Medical Center, 1400 Eighth Avenue, Fort Worth, TX 76104, USA
[b] Brookhaven Community College, 3939 Valley View Lane, Dallas, TX 75244, USA
* Corresponding author.
E-mail address: Margaret.McAtee@baylorhealth.edu (M. McAtee).

Crit Care Nurs Clin N Am 21 (2009) 391–401
doi:10.1016/j.ccell.2009.07.006   ccnursing.theclinics.com
0899-5885/09/$ – see front matter © 2009 Published by Elsevier Inc.

the height. Overweight is described as a BMI of 25 kg/m² or greater, obesity is described as a BMI or 30 kg/m², and severe or morbid obesity as a BMI of 40 kg/m². The World Health Organization has reported approximately 1.6 billion overweight adults and approximately 400 million who are obese. Further estimates indicate that by 2015, 2.3 billion adults will be overweight and 700 million will be obese.[3]

PATHOPHYSIOLOGY OF OBESITY

Adipose tissue is not just insulation around vital organs. Scientists have discovered that fat cells secrete a number of substances that help to regulate metabolic processes. These substances can also influence the patient's risk of developing other disorders including diabetes, hypertension, and atherosclerosis. These adipokines include adiponectin, leptin, interlukin-6 (IL-6), tumor necrosis factor-alpha (TNF-α), plasminogen activator-inhibitor-1 (PAI-1), resistin, and visfatin.[4] Adiponectin plays a part in glucose metabolism by affecting insulin sensitivity. It is also recognized as a biomarker for metabolic syndrome. Adiponectin may also act as an anti-inflammatory substance and protect against atherosclerosis. Low adiponectin levels are associated with an increased risk of diabetes mellitus type 2.[5] Although leptin acts as an appetite suppressant, obesity impairs this function and can lead to a resistance to leptin. In other words, the brain does not respond to the presence of leptin by controlling the appetite and the person continues to eat. The inflammatory proteins secreted by adipose tissue, including IL-6, TNF-α, and PAI-1, interfere with the ability of insulin to remove glucose from the blood stream. They also promote the development of atherosclerosis. PAI-1 along with fibrinogen can cause an increased risk of intravascular clotting. Resistin levels increase with increasing obesity and result in increased appetite, decrease in insulin sensitivity, and increased fat storage. Visfatin is a hormone with actions somewhat like insulin, but visfatin levels do not rise and fall in relationship to food intake.[4] Adiponectin exerts an anti-inflammatory effect, whereas resistin, leptin, and visfatin are proinflammatory.[6]

When assessing the elderly critically ill patient, height reduction that occurs with aging may influence the BMI. Also, geriatric patients tend to lose lean muscle mass and have more total body fat than their younger counterparts. Fat decreases in the arms and legs and increases in the trunk and abdomen.[7] For these patients, waist circumference may be a more reliable indicator of central obesity than BMI.[7]

RISKS AND PREVENTION STRATEGIES FOR THE PATIENT

One of the first questions that comes to the critical care nurse's mind when admitting an obese patient is, "What accommodations need to be made to safely care for this patient?" The answer encompasses equipment and environment, but also extends to additional observations and interventions, including psychosocial support. Because of the risks to obese patients, some institutions have developed multidisciplinary protocols for delivering care to bariatric patients.[7,8] The risks can be organized under the following headings: cardiovascular, pulmonary, nutritional, dermatologic, morbidity and mortality, gastrointestinal (GI), endocrine, immune, musculoskeletal, urinary, and pharmacologic. The cardiovascular, pulmonary, nutritional, dermatologic, and some of the pharmacologic risks related to sedation and pain management are covered elsewhere in this journal.

Morbidity and Mortality

Risk of mortality has been shown to increase as the BMI increases.[9,10] According to Cave and colleagues,[6] "obese critically ill patients have a more adverse outcome in a medical ICU compared with nonobese patients," although the mortality rate in critical care may not differ overall. In fact, the results of various studies provide conflicting information about the relationship of BMI to mortality in critically ill patients.[6,11,12] The increased adverse outcomes are probably a result of the comorbid conditions rather than obesity itself. Perhaps identifying and treating the risks of the associated pathologic conditions may protect against adverse outcomes and mortality. In any event, when the obese patient dies in critical care, extra large shrouds need to be available for postmortem care. The critical care nurse should also notify the mortuary of the patient's size so that the appropriate transport accommodations and mortuary equipment are available.[8]

Gastrointestinal

Obese patients have an enlarged abdomen that can cause increased abdominal pressure. If the patient is also diabetic, he or she may have gastroparesis. These two conditions can contribute to esophageal reflux which, in turn, places the patient at risk for aspiration with resultant lung injury.[13] Although GI prophylaxis with either a proton pump inhibitor or histamine$_2$ blocker should be considered for all critical care patients, obese patients are at an increased risk for complications if these medications are not used. Patient positioning, discussed elsewhere in this article, can be used to decrease the pressure of the abdominal wall on the stomach and diaphragm to minimize reflux as well. Measurement of abdominal girth from a marked site can be used to evaluate abdominal distention. Asking the patient if he or she is passing flatus is a more accurate method of assessing bowel function rather listening to bowel sounds.[14] Any patient receiving narcotics should be on a bowel regimen to avoid constipation. Obese patients, who have an increased abdominal girth to begin with, should be protected from straining to have a bowel movement.[15]

Endocrine

Central obesity, as measured by a waist circumference of 40 inches or more in men and 35 inches or more in women, contributes to metabolic syndrome, a disorder of insulin resistance (www.americanheart.org/presenter.jhtml?identifier=534). As discussed earlier, some of the substances secreted by adipose tissue, including resistin, IL-6, TNF-α, and PAI-1, interfere with glucose metabolism and contribute to insulin resistance.[4] Tight glycemic control (TGC) protocols have been introduced into ICUs as a best practice to improve clinical outcomes. Bariatric patients with insulin resistance may be resistant to the standard protocols. Joseph and colleagues[16] reported on a more aggressive insulin therapy protocol that demonstrated improved glycemic control without causing hypoglycemic episodes. Further studies may support the adoption of more intensive glucose control protocols. At any rate, critical care nurses need to be aware that obese patients require close monitoring and may need increased levels of insulin dosing to maintain glycemic control.

Immune

Obesity causes a low-level inflammatory response.[10] Release of proinflammatory proteins such as resistin, leptin, and visfatin help to maintain this state. When patients are admitted to the ICU, they are often experiencing another condition that also stimulates the immune response. Cave and colleagues[6] describe this as "the classic 1-hit-2-hit pattern of immune stimulation." This places the patient at increased risk for "organ failure, hyperglycemia, insulin resistance, infectious morbidity, longer ICU LOS, prolonged duration of mechanical ventilation, and greater mortality compared with their lean counterparts."[6] Interventions for the critical care nurse include monitoring white blood cell count, erythrocyte sedimentation rate, and C-reactive protein and maintaining tight glucose control.[17]

Musculoskeletal

Obesity places excessive strain on the musculoskeletal system. Disuse of muscles leads to deconditioning and muscle atrophy. Obese patients who are able should be encouraged to do active range of motion (ROM) exercises and to get out of bed with appropriate assistance. Those who are unable to move on their own should receive passive ROM as least once per shift to promote circulation and joint mobility. Obese patients may need a physical therapy or occupational therapy consult.[17]

Rhabdomyolysis can occur in any patient as a result of muscle compression and ischemia. Obese critically ill patients, especially if unconscious, have additional risks for rhabdomyolysis related to the difficulty in turning and positioning these patients. They may have had difficulty with mobility before being admitted to the hospital. Obese patients who undergo surgical procedures have an increased risk of developing rhabdomyolysis because of immobility and positioning during the operative procedure. Good assessment skills are critical in identifying this condition early so that interventions can be implemented to treat the patient and minimize complications. The critical care nurse should be suspicious of numbness or muscle pain in dependent parts. Brown urine may indicate the presence of myoglobin in the urine. Aggressive fluid replacement may be used to maintain intravascular volume.[18] These patients may also receive mannitol to mobilize fluid from the interstitial spaces and increase blood flow through the kidneys.[12]

Urinary

Obese patients may experience incontinence for a number of reasons. They may have difficulty using a standard size bedpan or bedside commode. If ambulatory, the standard hospital toilet in critical care may not be appropriate for them. If they need assistance in toileting, extra time is usually needed to ensure appropriate numbers of staff and transfer equipment to move the patient. The time delay may be too long and result in soiling themselves and the bed. The enlarged abdomen also places pressure on the bladder that may result in urgency and frequency. Some interventions strategies to prevent incontinence are to offer frequent toileting and to provide appropriately sized equipment. A large portable toilet seat that fits over a standard toilet may be useful for patients who can get out of bed. Good skin care is needed for patients experiencing incontinence paying special attention to skin folds in the lower abdomen and perineal area.[17]

A urinary catheter may be necessary for frequent or urgent monitoring of urinary output, inability to void because of neurogenic bladder, to prevent skin breakdown, or to protect a wound in the perineal or sacral area.[19] When placing a urinary catheter, three staff members may be needed for insertion. For female patients, two staff members should position the legs and retract the labial folds while a third person preps the perineal area and inserts the catheter. When inserting a catheter in a male patient, two staff members may be needed to lift the abdominal folds so that the penis can be exposed for the third member to prep and insert the catheter.[13]

Vascular Access

Obtaining and maintaining reliable vascular access is an important consideration for any critical care patient. The obese patient presents a challenge. Increased amounts of subcutaneous adipose tissue can obscure the usual landmarks making it difficult to place peripheral intravenous catheters. In addition, the catheters may need to be longer to penetrate the greater subcutaneous tissue mass and be placed securely in the vein and the angle of insertion may need to be different.[8,12] Central venous catheters may be necessary. Use of the internal jugular vein may provide the best site with fewest complications.[12]

Pharmacologic

Pharmacokinetics includes the absorption, distribution, metabolism, and excretion of medications. Pharmacokinetics of particular medications may be altered in the setting of obesity, especially distribution and excretion.[20] Greater amounts of adipose tissue suggest the need to administer increased doses of lipophilic medications to achieve the desired effect, but the half life of these medications may be prolonged because of the increased medication stored in adipose tissue. Obese patients with normal renal function may demonstrate an increased rate of clearance for drugs excreted by the kidney because of an increased glomerular filtration rate related to increased kidney mass.[12] Many of the drugs given within the critical care setting have recommendations to adjust the dose according to the patient's weight. However, very few studies have evaluated the dosing of medications in obese and morbidly obese patients. Even lean individuals exhibit a wide variation in serum concentrations of many drugs commonly used in critical care.[21]

Consultation with a pharmacist is indicated because of the complexity of determining appropriate dosing of medications for critically ill obese patients.[8,18] With some medications, weight-based dosing is not indicated. In others, ideal body weight (IBW) may be the appropriate measure. Still others may require an adjusted weight based on ideal body weight and a percentage of excess body weight over and above ideal body weight. This may be termed the dosing weight (DW).[20,21] Intravenous medication use avoids the issue of distribution but not renal clearance. Use of other forms of medication administration, including topical, intramuscular, and subcutaneous injections, results in unpredictable rates of absorption because of poor perfusion to fatty tissue.[13,18]

Dosing of many of the medications used in critical care may be guided by serum levels of the drug or other assays. For some of these medications, the initial dose may be calculated using IBW or DW. After results of serum levels are available, dosing can be adjusted for the individual. In the case of anticoagulation, unfractionated heparin (UFH) may be preferable to low molecular weight heparin (LMWH) for several reasons. Heparin can be given intravenously with dosing guided by activated partial thromboplastin time (aPTT) results. LMWHs, on the other hand, are given subcutaneously resulting in unpredictable absorption and distribution. Dosing may be guided by anti-factor Xa heparin assay (anti-Xa) monitoring, but this is not readily available in all settings.[21]

Critical care nurses often initiate vasoactive drips. Little information exists on weight-based dosing of these medications. Whether to use an IBW or actual body weight depends on the indication and urgency of the patient situation. A conservative approach may be best. In this case, the nurse may choose to use IBW and then titrate the medication based on the patient's response.[21,22]

RISKS AND PREVENTION STRATEGIES FOR CRITICAL CARE NURSES

Morbidly obese patients are often associated with a higher risk of comorbidities and therefore have a higher incidence of being admitted to the critical care unit. These patients can be challenging, as even routine care can be complicated by their size alone. Complications in caring for the morbidly obese patient, however, are not complications for the patient alone. Along with these complications come increased risks for staff. The most common injury to the staff caring for the morbidly obese critical care patient is low back injury. Low back injuries can be up to 70% of the injuries to staff as a result of transferring, lifting, and positioning the morbidly obese patient. In addition to low back injuries there are also reports of upper extremity, shoulder, and neck injuries.

As with any risk, the more exposure to the causative factor, the greater the chance the risk will become a reality. Increased exposure to risk for injury, while caring for the obese patient, is the actual increased workload of the staff delivering the care. Risks that are impacted by the increased workload include the patient's pain level, the patient's fear of falling, equipment availability and procurement, resource allocation of staff, staff attitude toward caring for the morbidly obese patient, and environmental challenges.

RISK FOR STAFF INJURY: MOVING THE PATIENT

The patient's pain level can be correlated with his or her inability to assist in any movement.[23] Injuries have been associated with the direct workload of caring for these patients.[23] When a patient is in pain, it is more difficult for him or her to be able to assist in moving and can even result in resistance to move. This resistance or hesitation to move results in increasing the caregiver's workload and risk for injury while transferring or positioning these patients.

A patient's fear of falling will decrease his or her confidence in moving, even with the assistance of lift equipment. Obese patients are fearful the equipment will not be strong enough to hold them and may pull back or withdraw. The fear interferes with the patient's ability to assist in moving, transferring, or ambulating. Patients are reluctant to move forward or initiate movement for fear of loosing balance, breaking equipment, and falling. This reluctance will further increase the caregiver workload in assisting the patient, resulting in a higher risk of injury to the caregiver.[24]

Availability and procurement of proper lift and transfer equipment is critical to avoid staff injury. Trying to move a morbidly obese patient without lift equipment is not only dangerous for the staff, but also for the patient. Frequently the equipment is ordered by size alone but is not always effective in supporting the obese patient.[23] All needed equipment is not always available. Some or part of the equipment may be accessible. Equipment needed includes but is not limited to specialized bariatric bed systems, patient transport and lift devices, bariatric turning and repositioning slings, floor-mounted toilets, and walkers.

STAFFING REQUIREMENTS

Improper size or the lack of appropriate equipment is not the only risk for staff injury in working with the morbidly obese patients. A lack of the appropriate number of staff on duty can result in an increased workload for those who are working, resulting in potential or real staff injuries. There are estimates as high as needing twice as many staff to complete a simple activity such as bathing the morbidly obese patient.[25] The need can be as high as five staff members to provide safe lifting; one for monitoring the airway, one at the head, one on each side, and one at the foot. Five staff members could be all the unit staff available on a shift. Requiring all available staff to deliver care to one patient takes time and attention from other patients, resulting in risk exposure for those patients also.

Staffing resources are also a factor in transporting the obese patient from the patient care unit to other areas of the hospital. Tests and procedures are not always scheduled Monday through Friday on the day shift. Other areas in the hospital often decrease their staff after hours and on weekends. When an obese patient requires a trip to radiology on the night shift, there are fewer hospital resources during those hours to assist in the transport or monitoring in those areas. Timing of required off-unit services becomes crucial in finding assistance to simply take an obese patient for an x-ray.

NURSES' ATTITUDES TOWARD THE OBESE PATIENT

Nurses' attitudes toward the morbidly obese is reported to range from negativity, blaming the patient for his or her own state, to that of personal sacrifice for the care of the patient.[26] The difference in attitudes can be attributed to a difference in age of the caregiver. Younger nurses are more of the persuasion that it is the patients' own lack of control that has lead to their obesity and they should be held accountable for their actions or lack of self control to loose weight. Older nurses have been reported as believing if the patient has a need to be moved or repositioned, it is the nurse's responsibility to see that the patient is moved, even at the risk of self-injury.[24] These nurses believe it is their duty to provide for their patients, no matter the cost to them personally, even if there is a lack of equipment or other staff members to assist them.

HOSPITAL ENVIRONMENT

Moving the obese patient is not limited to turning or positioning. These patients are frequently required to move throughout the facility. They are admitted from the Emergency Department, front lobby, or even day surgery and travel through the operating room, radiology, CT scanner, or other diagnostic or treatment areas. The environment is not always obese friendly to caregivers facilitating the transport. Elevators with narrow doors, ceilings without lifts, even doorways too small for the bariatric bed to pass through can be dangerous for caregivers to navigate, increasing their workload. Critical care nurses are often left to their own creativity in improvising ways to move these patients from area to area, leading to an increased risk of injury to both caregivers and patients.

PREVENTION STRATEGIES
Pain Management

Managing the patient's pain level allows more comfort for the patient to assist with moving and positioning. Increasing the patient's comfort and ability to assist in movement will decrease the caregiver's exposure to additional lifting. Getting patients comfortable allows them more confidence in being able to assist with moving and transferring. If it hurts less when they move, the more apt they are to do so, decreasing the caregiver's workload and risk for injury. Sleep apnea and respiratory difficulties are common in the obese patients. Therefore, patient-controlled analgesia (PCA) pumps are the pain management choice of most surgeons. PCA pumps allow patients to control their own medication delivery rate, providing additional safety from oversedation and decreased respiratory effort.[24]

Equipment

Supporting the patient with the appropriate weight capacity equipment and well-fitted slings will provide a greater sense of security for the patient while decreasing workload and risk exposure for the caregiver. Obese patients' fear of falling, not knowing if the apparatus chosen to move them will hold their weight, hampers their ability to relax, to assist with moving, and to reduce reluctance to moving. Equipment must be safe, properly sized, and provide the appropriate amount of support in moving obese patients. Patient and family education regarding safety of equipment to be used also decreases patient anxiety and resistance. If they understand how the equipment works and the weight capacity of the equipment, any reluctance to allow the use of the equipment decreases.[24]

Procurement of the proper equipment must include staff input. Critical care nurses are more likely to buy into and use equipment if they have been included in the selection process. Successful programs for safe patient handling must include staff recommendations.[13] Equipment must be selected based on the weight capacity, not just by ordering an extra large size. The most common bariatric equipment selection is the patient bed. The bed must not only be able to hold the increased weight, but also be able to help in positioning, providing pressure relief, and decreasing the risk of decubitus.[24] Bariatric bed systems are available to accommodate up to 1000 pounds and can be designed to assist with turning, positioning, and pressure-relief therapy. In addition to the bed itself, proper lift and transfer devices must be readily available to move the patient to and from the bed. These devices can be portable or mounted from the ceiling and, just as with the bed, must have the appropriate weight capacity.

Staffing Resources

To provide safe adequate staffing resources for nursing units caring for morbidly obese patients there must also be a mechanism to measure and quantify the increased workload these patients require. Even simple tasks such as bathing have been observed as requiring up to five staff members.[27] Procurement of staff must be planned well in advance to ensure the availability of an increased number of staff, just as in ensuring the availability of needed equipment. One such approach to ensuring the availability and correct measurement of staff is to cohort the obese patients in the same unit. Having a specific area or unit these patients are admitted to can ensure not only the appropriate equipment availability, but also the correct numbers of staff prepared to care for them.[24]

Staffing resources, however, should not be limited to a specific number of personnel only. Other resources that should be available to the staff include techniques in lifting; lift teams, ergonomic training, safety committees, and patient care planning to inform other caregivers of successful safe patient handling. These resources can assist in providing training to a consistent team of caregivers using the equipment, minimizing risks to specific areas that are most prepared to provide care, and controlling risk exposure.[13]

Sensitivity Training for Critical Care Nurses

Staff attitudes toward the obese patient, whether negative toward the patient, or believing the patient must be cared for no matter the risk for the caregiver, both increase the stress in caring for these patients and increase the workload in doing so. Tools that must be provided for all staff caring for these patients include sensitivity training. Staff must be aware that patient dignity and self-esteem must be preserved while at the same time using heavy equipment and additional personnel to swing them through the air in a large sling suspended from the ceiling. Sensitivity training can also include approaches to communicating with patients and families, in addition to how to support and assist each other. Caregivers must be trained in how to encourage the patient to develop trust in equipment and techniques that will assist them in their care. Training must be given in how to develop nurse-to-nurse consulting in uses of equipment and ergonomic techniques and that it is appropriate to ask for help critical to reducing workload. Activating and participating in safe patient handling teams is also a resource available and appropriate to access to decrease stress and workload. Providing care for the morbidly obese patient can often resemble an emotional roller coaster of stress, not only for the patients, but also for the caregivers. The stress, however, can be decreased for all by adequate and consistent sensitivity training.

HOSPITAL ENVIRONMENT

Numbers of staff, physician orders for pharmaceutical agents, appropriate equipment, correct sizing of slings, and staff sensitivity are all resources manageable by planning, ordering, and training. More difficult are the sometimes tricky environmental challenges. Narrow doors, small elevators, inadequate operating rooms, and expensive radiology equipment are not so easily corrected to make the environment morbidly obese friendly. Moving and transferring the obese patient throughout the hospital often presents unique obstacles. To overcome these obstacles, staff must plan ahead, plot alternate routes, and engage the help of facility operations and maintenance personnel. It may be necessary to rent some equipment, ie, operating room tables, equipment, or instruments to meet the needs of obese patients. As the prevalence of morbidly obese patients increases, hospitals must allow for these increased needs when planning any expansion, construction, or procurement of expensive radiology equipment such as CT scanners, MRI machines, or nuclear medicine suites. These increased needs have an increased crunch on hospital capital funding and sometimes even the survivability of programs.

Everyday caregivers are at an increasing risk for physical injury in caring for the increasing number of morbidly obese patients admitted to the hospital with increasing BMIs and increasing comorbidities. Risk factors and prevention strategies have been identified. Caregivers must work together with health care facilities to recognize, address, and ensure there is ongoing collaboration to implement the prevention strategies and protect caregivers from unnecessary injuries.

SUMMARY

As the number of obese people in this country increases, more and more patients admitted to critical care units are obese or morbidly obese. Critical care nurses need to understand what makes these patients different from people of normal size and those who are merely overweight. Obese and morbidly obese patients have increased risks of problems when admitted to the critical care environment. Critical care nurse are also at increased risk when caring for these patients. Identification of risks to both patients and nurses has been identified as well as recommendations to address those risks. More research is needed to understand fully changes that should be made in critical care units so that appropriate care is delivered to optimize patient outcomes and promote safety for critically ill obese patients and critical care nurses.

REFERENCES

1. Centers for Disease Control. Obesity: halting the epidemic by making health easier. Available at: http://www.cdc.gov/NCCDPHP/publications/AAG/obesity. htm. Accessed March 8, 2009.
2. Weight-control Information Network. Statistics related to overweight and obesity. Available at: http://win.niddk.nih.gov/statistics/index.htm. Accessed March 8, 2009.

3. World Health Organization. Obesity and overweight. Available at: http://www.who.int/infobase. Accessed March 8, 2009.

4. Etienne MO, Pavlovich-Danis SJ. Body fat shapes patients' health. Available at: https://lms.nurse.com/PrintTopics.aspx?topicid=1034. Accessed December 30, 2008.

5. Ley S, Harris S, Connelly P, et al. Adipokines and incident type 2 diabetes in a Canadian Aborigine population: the sandy lake health and diabetes project. Diabetes Care 2008;31(7):1410–5.

6. Cave M, Hurt R, Frazier T, et al. Obesity, inflammation, and the potential application of pharmaconutrition. Nutr Clin Pract 2008;23(1):16–34.

7. Arzouman J, Lacovara J, Blackett A, et al. Developing a comprehensive bariatric protocol: a template for improving patient care. Medsurg Nurs 2006;15(1):21–6.

8. Hurst S, Blanco K, Boyle D, et al. Bariatric implications of critical care nursing. Dimens Crit Care Nurs 2004;23(2):76–83.

9. Ray D, Matchett S, Baker K, et al. The effect of body mass index on patient outcomes in a medical ICU. Chest 2005;127(6):2125–31.

10. Vachharajani V, Vital S. Obesity and sepsis. J Intensive Care Med 2006;21(5):287–95.

11. Goulenok C, Monchi M, Chiche J, et al. Influence of overweight on ICU mortality: a prospective study. Chest 2004;125(4):1441–5.

12. Pieracci F, Barie P, Pomp A. Critical care of the bariatric patient. Crit Care Med 2006;34(6):1796–804.

13. Ide P, Farber E, Lautz D. Perioperative nursing care of the bariatric surgical patient. AORN J 2008;88(1):30–58.

14. Harrington L. Postoperative care of patients undergoing bariatric surgery. Medsurg Nurs 2006;15(6):357–63.

15. Wilson J, Clark J. Obesity: impediment to wound healing. Crit Care Nurs Q 2003;26(2):119–32.

16. Joseph B, Genaw J, Carlin A, et al. Perioperative tight glycemic control: the challenge of bariatric surgery patients and the fear of hypoglycemic events. The Permanente Journal 2007;11(2). Available at: http://xnet.kp.org/permanentejournal/spring07/perioperative.html. Accessed March 23, 2009.

17. Harris H. Nursing care of the morbidly obese patient. Nursing Made Incredibly Easy 2008;6(3):34–43.

18. Barth M, Jenson C. Postoperative nursing care of gastric bypass patients. Am J Crit Care 2006;15(4):378–88.

19. DuBeau C. Champ: bedside teaching: indications for Foley catheter use. Available at: http://pritzker.bsd.uchicago.edu/CHAMP/Trigger_IndicationsforFoleyCathUse_8_3_04FINALCD.pdf. Accessed March 15, 2009.

20. Davidson J, Kruse M, Cox D, et al. Critical care of the morbidly obese. Crit Care Nurs Q 2003;26(2):105–18.

21. Erstad BL. Dosing of medications in morbidly obese patients in the intensive care unit setting. Intensive Care Med 2004;30(1):18–32.

22. Harrington L. Ask the experts. Crit Care Nurse 2006;26(5):68–71.

23. United States Department of Veterans Affairs. Safe bariatric patient handling toolkit. Available at: www.visn8.med.va.gov/patientsafetycenter. Accessed January 14, 2009.

24. Baptiste A, Leffard B, Vieira E, et al. Roundtable discussion. Caregiver injury and safe patient handling. Bariatric Nursing and Surgical Patient Care 2007;2(1):7–16.

25. Rose M, Baker G, Drake D, et al. A comparison of nurse staffing requirements for the care of morbidly obese and non-obese patients in the acute care setting. Bariatric Nursing and Surgical Patient Care 2007;2(1):53–6.

26. Brown I. Nurses' attitudes towards adult patients who are obese: literature review. J Adv Nurs 2006;53(2):221–32.

27. Rose M, Baker G, Drake D, et al. Nurse staffing requirements for care of morbidly obese patients in the acute care setting. Bariatric Nursing and Surgical Patient Care 2006;1(2):115–21.

The Impact of Obesity on Critical Care Resource Use and Outcomes

Chris Winkelman, RN, PhD, CCRN, ACNP[a],*,
Beverly Maloney, RN, MSN, APRN, CCRN[b], Janet Kloos, RN, PhD, CNS, CCRN[c]

KEYWORDS

• Obese • Critically ill • Resources • Outcomes • ICU

Annually, more than 5 million adults are admitted to an ICU.[1] Reports indicate that 12% to 37% of adult patients admitted to an ICU are obese.[2–7] Obese patients in the ICU present unique challenges to the health care team and specific challenges to nurses. This article reviews the science and art of resource use for obese patients in the ICU. Staff nurses and advanced practice nurses (APNs) can make important contributions to improving outcomes in this population of unique and vulnerable patients.

Variations in weight and body mass index (BMI) have implications for drug and nutrition management. At the bedside, however, it is not the absolute weight or source of weight (eg, adipose tissue, muscle, temporary water weight; or fat distribution at the hip or waist), but the body habitus that impacts nursing care. Patients who have a large body size require special equipment, additional time and personnel for procedures, special monitoring and surveillance, and modified interventions for routine care. These patients also are at increased risk for complications and adverse outcomes related to critical illness. For the purposes of this article, "obesity" is defined as a large BMI (ie, > 30 kg/m^2) or, simply, as a very large body size.

RESOURCE USE

For this article, "resource use" refers to adjustments to common approaches to monitoring and interventions, requisite equipment, and use of personnel to provide direct care. A review of the literature and experience suggests that many adjustments to resource use occur during planning and implementing ICU care for obese patients.

[a] Frances Payne Bolton School of Nursing, Case Western Reserve University, 10900 Euclid Ave, Cleveland, OH 44106, USA
[b] Fairview Hospital CCHS, 18101 Lorain Road, Cleveland, OH 44111, USA
[c] University Hospitals, Case Medical Center, 11100 Euclid Avenue, Cleveland, OH 44106, USA
* Corresponding author.
E-mail address: chris.winkelman@case.edu (C. Winkelman).

Crit Care Nurs Clin N Am 21 (2009) 403–422
doi:10.1016/j.ccell.2009.07.002   ccnursing.theclinics.com
0899-5885/09/$ – see front matter © 2009 Elsevier Inc. All rights reserved.

For example, the ability to monitor and the need to focus surveillance on unique risks alters nursing practice at the bedside: placing ECG leads, using skin care products, and applying a blood pressure cuff require variations in typical practice routines. There are few studies about resource use among critically ill obese adults. Most data for guiding care in the ICU are observational. There are no standard guidelines, although individual expert opinions have been published.[8–11] When there is evidence to support an intervention, it is graded as either "A" (from a randomized, controlled trial or meta-analysis) or "B" (evidence from other sources, such as uncontrolled studies).

Monitoring and Special Care Considerations

Vigilance to prevent respiratory failure and skin breakdown consume ICU nursing time with obese patients. Comorbidities in this population often increase the need for monitoring and modified surveillance. Data-driven interventions focus on the pulmonary system and adjustments to monitoring. Obese critically ill patients are twice as likely to suffer a critical respiratory event such as unanticipated hypoxemia, hypoventilation, or upper airway obstruction requiring an intervention than nonobese patients in a post-anesthesia care unit (PACU) (evidence grade B).[12] When respiratory problems occur in a PACU, admission to the ICU is likely.[11] Morbidly obese patients spend more time mechanically ventilated and require more oxygen during hospitalization.[3] Recognizing and treating obstructive sleep apnea may prevent respiratory failure and is recommended as part of preoperative evaluation in obese patients (evidence grade B).[11,13] In addition, the number of comorbidities may place the obese patient at risk for injury or complications; vigilance regarding changes in cardiac and pulmonary status is essential to detect adverse changes early and to avoid failure to rescue. Frequent monitoring and surveillance can delay transfer from the ICU to reduce risk and complications related to airway, breathing, or circulation compromise.

The use of noninvasive mechanical ventilation (NIMV) to support ventilatory effort, especially during sleep, is recommended for obese patients diagnosed with obstructive sleep apnea. Providing oral hygiene has not been specifically examined in patients receiving NIMV, but data extrapolated from mechanically ventilated patients suggests that oral hygiene can reduce iatrogenic pneumonia and promote comfort.[14] For patients receiving NIMV, measures to promote mouth decontamination may not relieve the discomfort commonly experienced with high-flow air during NIMV. In the authors' experience, patients with face masks for NIMV frequently complain about mouth dryness. One strategy to provide optimal care is to follow an oral hygiene schedule but to supplement the scheduled decontamination interventions with artificial saliva or other products. Adding humidification to airflow also may alleviate discomfort. A dry mouth not only is uncomfortable but may contribute to drying of mucus, so that increased effort is required for airway clearance, and to mucosal or lip injury. Diseases such as sarcoidosis and other autoimmune conditions and medications such as anticholinergics can contribute to oral dryness. Some agents that can be used (but not substituted for brushing, chlorhexidine, or other decontaminating regimens) are Biotene and Oral Balance. These products contain salivary enzymes (ie, lactoperoxidase, glucose oxidase, and lysozyme) that interact with oral bacterial systems. Also, carboxymethyl or hydroxyethylcellulous solutions such as Optimoist, Entertainer's Secret, Oralube, and Saliva Substitute are available as over-the-counter products.[15] One practice guideline suggests using petroleum jelly on the lips and one of the hydrating agents every 2 to 4 hours, although there are no specific empiric data to support the frequency or type of hydrating agent.[16]

Surveillance to detect early changes in respiratory health such as assessing breath sounds and heart sounds is difficult. Assisting the patient to a side-lying position for auscultation of posterior breath sounds may be easier than requesting the patient to sit forward when the abdominal size is large. End-tidal monitoring for carbon dioxide may not be reliable in obese patients because of their wide arterial–alveolar gradients (grade B).[9] Attention to subtle signs of increasing carbon dioxide levels such as changes in cognition, consciousness, and restlessness/restfulness are incorporated into assessment routines.

The morbidly obese patient is at increased risk for skin irritation, odor, and break-down within skin folds that trap perspiration.[17] Fungal infections often occur because of this moisture within the folds. The obese patient also is prone to cellulitis from decreased circulation, immune system compromise, and the hyperglycemia from co-morbid diabetes. In addition to the regular causes of skin injury, atypical pressure injuries can occur from the use of standard hospital equipment because of pressure on hips from too narrow chairs or pressure on arms from the side rails of a too narrow bed. Placing the patient in a bed designed for the obese helps prevent skin break-down, because bariatric beds are equipped with special mattresses to prevent pres-sure injury and are wider than the average bed. One should assess the skin in an anterior position by examining skin between folds, under breasts, in the axillary region, and all along pannus. With the patient in the side-lying position, visualize the back, buttocks, and neck. Identify areas with moisture, redness, excoriation, or evidence of yeast infection and intervene immediately. Be sure that skin between folds is dry after bathing. Avoid powder, because it is made from ground limestone; powder is abrasive and tends to clump, especially within skin folds. Moisture in skin folds can be absorbed by abdominal pads or by commercial products such as Interdry Ag, which wicks the moisture to outside the skin fold and contains silver to treat any infec-tious agents present. Extra personnel may be needed to lift pannus and/or skin folds to visualize skin adequately. For patients who are admitted with pressure ulcers or skin tears, ask the patient or family about the circumstances related to the wound devel-opment and obtain their evaluation about the current status. Ask about products that have been used successfully. Tape may contribute to skin breakdown; consider the use of alternate anchoring devices in moist, fragile skin.

Monitoring cardiac rhythm is challenging. Increased chest size obscures anatomic landmarks for lead placement. Variable lead placement prevents early recognition of ST waveform changes and alters the characteristics of waveforms for alarm triggers and dysrhythmia analysis. Accurate lead placement is essential, and guidelines for finding anatomic landmarks must be used for accurate diag-nosis.[18,19] Identify landmarks with indelible markers and prepare skin for efficient operation of electrodes.

Obtaining a noninvasive blood-pressure measurement often requires special equip-ment or positioning regular equipment on alternate sites. A large or extra-large cuff may be needed for the upper arm, but the shape of the upper arm often means that the large or extra-large cuff does not fit snugly or end 2 to 3 cm above the antecubital fossa. A regular cuff on the forearm can provide consistent readings (evidence grade A).[20] When using a forearm measurement, be sure the forearm is at heart level to main-tain reliability and validity of the reading. A calf pressure also may be used in the obese patient. For all cuff measurements of blood pressure, the cuff must have a bladder large enough encircle 80% of the limb.[20]

There are no data to suggest that unique laboratory testing is needed routinely for obese patients while in the ICU, but more frequent monitoring of drug levels or eval-uation of toxicity (eg, renal or liver function) must be considered when administering antibiotics, anticoagulants, sedatives, opioids and insulin (no evidence grade).[21] Obese patients may be at increased risk for rhabdomyolysis after prolonged immobility, resulting in additional laboratory evaluation when clinically indicated (evidence grade B).[22]

Positioning and Mobility

Patients in the ICU often need assistance with positioning in bed. Even with special mattresses, it is recommended that repositioning for comfort, lung expansion, and inspection of skin integrity occur every 2 hours for all patients (evidence grade B). A full-body lateral rotation support surface on a bariatric bed can be used as an adjunct for turning and repositioning obese patients. While the patient is in bed, a reverse Trendelenburg position improves the mechanics of breathing in a patient who has a large abdomen as compared with a chair position with hips flexed (evidence grade B).[23] After extubation, increased intra-abdominal pressure and weight from thoracic fat can restrict lung and diaphragmatic excursion and impair the patient's ability to clear the airway. Therefore bedside suctioning should be provided, along with frequent surveillance, coaching for deep breathing, and assistance with coughing to maintain airway and oxygenation during spontaneous respirations (no evidence grade).

A lateral transfer to a stretcher or cart is best accomplished with a sliding board, an air-assisted friction-reducing device, or a mechanical lift when the patient cannot assist. If the patient is transferring from bed to chair, there are seating transfer aids (eg, assisting chair-to-chair or chair-to-commode transfers), bariatric stand assist lifts, and full-body slings that can be used. Newer bariatric full-body slings are easier to place than older models, requiring less effort from both patient and staff so that energy can be used for the actual out-of-bed transfer. The typical lift aids used in the ICU have a weight limit. Specialty mobilizing devices for the morbidly obese patient are listed in Appendix 1. Because obese patients may be at increased risk for rhabdomyolysis during prolonged immobility, a plan for early, progressive mobility must be considered and evaluated daily. If ramps are present, provide additional personnel when transferring from the emergency department to the ICU or from the ICU to another unit so that extra help will be available to push on upward slopes or to slow down the cart or bed on downward slopes.

Guidelines for preventing staff injury during positioning and mobility interventions indicate that the maximum weight a nurse should lift is about 35 lb (no evidence grade; expert opinion).[24] Back injuries are common in health care and account for more than 24% of all occupational injuries and illnesses involving days away from work.[25] Considering the safety needs of staff is important before implementing out-of-bed activity for all patients.[26] During any patient-handling intervention, when a caregiver is required to lift more than 35 lb of a patient's weight, the patient should be considered dependent, and an assistive device should be used. Other resources that help mobilize obese patients are wide chairs or benches. Even with assistive devices, multiple caregivers will be needed to move or reposition an obese patient.

Algorithms for safe patient handling developed by expert clinicians in conjunction with ergomatic specialists are available for testing and implementation (www.visn8. med.va.gov/patientsafetycenter/).[24] These algorithms advocate early progressive mobility and describe techniques and equipment that promote safe patient movement. Specific algorithms for the obese or bariatric patient include in-bed and out-of bed guides to care. On the Web site, there is an associated curriculum to teach techniques for safe patient handling.[24]

Environment of Care: Equipment, Procedural Time, and Transportation

Unique temporary and permanent equipment is needed to provide care for the obese ICU patient. Large beds, gowns, wheelchairs, and blood pressure cuffs are needed to provide care. Doorframes need to be wider so larger bed frames can be moved in and out of rooms. Toilets mounted to the floor are safer than wall-mounted commodes. Longer surgical gloves and needles may be needed to treat larger patients. Larger shrouds and communication with the morgue may be needed in the case of death.

There are technical challenges in line placement and securing devices when the critically ill patient is obese. For example, large neck circumference seems to predict difficult intubation and also requires a longer tracheal tube when tracheotomy is performed.[27] Standard tracheostomy tubes usually are too curved and too short to fit properly because of the increased distance to the trachea in the obese patient. Several studies report increased major and minor complications during percutaneous tracheostomy, including major complications such as bleeding or malpositioning and minor events such as hypoxia and subcutaneous emphysema (evidence grade B).[28–32] In these reports, morbid obesity is more likely to be associated with adverse outcomes during tracheotomy procedures, but obesity does not lead to an increased incidence of tracheotomy (evidence grade B).[28,33] Care of the obese patient after tracheostomy is similar to that for normal-weight patients: patients need careful and frequent assessment to ensure that sutures and devices that hold the tracheostomy tube in place do not irritate or erode skin.

Line placement into a central vein can be challenging without visible anatomic landmarks and with decreased neck mobility in morbidly obese ICU patients. In addition, finding pulses and using ultrasound to guide insertion may be more difficult for both venous and arterial line placement, and line placement may require more time. Some authors suggest using a longer line or needle for insertion. Similarly, while administering an intramuscular injection, one should compress the fatty subcutaneous layer with one hand or use a longer needle. Securing lines and maintaining a sterile dressing at the neck also is problematic and may require a nonstandard occlusive dressing.

Another resource-intensive procedure is imaging in obese ICU patients. In one 15-year retrospective study, about 750,000 radiologic examinations included the disclaimer "limited by body habitus."[34] As many as 10% to 15% of hospitalized patients may not be able to be imaged because of equipment limitations.[35] Plain radiograph, ultrasound, and nuclear medicine images are all attenuated by body fat. Increased radiation is needed with radiographs in obese individuals. Multiple cassettes may be needed to cover the chest or abdominal views of an obese individual, with additional exposure to x-rays. Radioisotopes are dosed by weight; obese patients may exceed the maximum dose, decreasing the quality of nuclear medicine images.[34] A CT table can hold 700 lb, but the table motor can fail with a 350- to 380-lb load.[8] New operating room and diagnostic tables in x-ray are designed to hold 700 lb rather than the more typical 350 lb of older models. There are additional limitations from the gantry (ie, opening) diameter; older models have an aperture of about 70 cm, which is reduced by 15 to 18 cm when the table is advanced. A waist or chest circumference greater than 130 inches will not fit. The table limits for most MRI with open-field scanners is 550 lb. The larger cross-sectional area to be imaged in obese patients requires increased scan times, which may lead to more motion artifact or increased risk for airway or ventilatory compromise from prolonged supine positioning. Finally, interventional radiology such as radiofrequency ablation or stent placement may not be available to obese patients in the radiology department because of equipment limitations and reduced image quality.

A recurring theme in the data related to procedural time and equipment is differences between obese patients and morbidly obese patients. When empiric data are analyzed, patients who have a BMI greater than 40 kg/m^2 are more likely to need more time, expertise, and equipment than patients who have a BMI less than 39.99 kg/m^2. Again, it is not BMI but body size and body characteristics such as neck circumference that are likely to influence clinical decisions in the care of the obese, critically ill patient.

Nutrition

Nutrition is essential therapy in all critically ill adults. The advantages of early enteral nutrition for patients receiving mechanical ventilation or diagnosed with brain injury, burns, or surgery include reduced length of stay (LOS), decreased infection, improved function, and fewer wound complications (evidence grade A).[36,37] Current consensus in the literature is to provide 60% of caloric needs with sufficient protein to preserve lean mass and avoid consumption of visceral proteins in obese, critically ill adult patients (evidence grade B).[36,38–40] Permissive underfeeding does not jeopardize immune function or wound healing and can promote weight loss.[36,41]

Obese patients may have more risk for aspiration with supine positioning during enteral feeding with concurrent intubation. Obese patients have increased intra-abdominal pressure from subcutaneous and visceral adipose deposits. ICU nurses need to be vigilant in providing backrest elevation greater than 30° to reduce aspiration risk. As well, assessment for enteral feeding intolerance including evaluation of residual volume and gastrointestinal symptoms (eg, nausea, distension, and emesis) may need adjustment in this population. In the ICU, enteral feedings usually are not stopped until two residuals of 200 to 250 mL over 1 to 2 hours are determined by the bedside nurse.[42] Adjustments for the obese patient may include more frequent monitoring with smaller residuals of 100 to 200 mL. Increased intra-abdominal pressure may contribute to more frequent or larger aspiration volumes in the presence of relatively small residuals.[43]

Insulin regimens for glycemic control, especially during nutrition therapy, also may require more resources. Insulin resistance is common among obese individuals. Changes in both pharmacokinetics and pharmacodynamics of insulin during acute and critical illness may require larger doses or increased frequency of administration. With the uncertain absorption of subcutaneously administered insulin in obese patients with peripheral fluid redistribution, achieving glycemic control may be particularly problematic in the ICU setting when intravenous routes are not used.

Adjustments in Drug Use

Obesity may increase the risk of therapeutic failure or drug toxicity. There is limited information about the pharmacokinetics of drugs common in the ICU setting; most drugs are studied in outpatient or community settings. Generally, both distribution and clearance of drugs are likely to be altered by obesity. Clearance can be increased in obese individuals who have normal renal function, a phenomenon that is attributed to a larger kidney mass (evidence grade B).[44] Distribution can be affected by the chemical properties of drugs; lipophilic drugs are distributed to adipose tissue. Greater adiposity may mean a larger dose is needed to achieve a therapeutic serum or tissue level. Drugs with a high volume of distribution (ie, lipophilic drugs) can be adjusted during a loading dose based on total body weight; drugs with a smaller distribution factor are loaded based on lean body weight. For many drugs, there is a cap on the dose so that obese patients receive either a maximum recommended dose or a dose based on adjusted body weight rather than on actual weight.

Altered distribution in obesity can affect duration of effect. Prolonged administration of lipophilic drugs can result in deposition in adipose tissue; the stored drug is released slowly, causing ongoing effects even after cessation of the drug. In addition, the mode of administration can affect drug onset and effects. Drugs given transdermally or subcutaneously are likely to have variable absorption because of the reduced vascularity of adipose tissue compared with dermis, fascia, or muscle tissue. Poor absorption can lead to unpredictable drug onset and duration.44 Suggestions for dosing obese patients with some antibiotics, heparin, opioids, and sedatives have been developed based on expert opinion and case control studies (evidence grade B).[44]

Effective dosing ranges for many anti-infective agents have not been examined specifically in critically ill obese patients. Because many antibiotics are hydrophilic and are not widely distributed, sufficient blood levels are thought to be achievable at recommended doses. In the case of anti-infectives including quinolones, cephalosporins, and carbapenums, dosing at the high end of treatment ranges is recommended, especially in severely obese patients who have symptomatic infections.[45] Both aminoglycosides and vancomycin are somewhat lipophilic, so effectiveness and renal function may need close monitoring in severely obese patients.[46] More frequent administration of aminoglycosides and vancomycin, rather than a single daily dose schedule, is advised to achieve therapeutic blood levels while avoiding toxicities.[45] Data from healthy, obese adults suggest that modifying the dose of an aminoglycoside based on the calculation of adjusted body weight rather than actual or ideal body weight is reasonable.[45] Prophylaxis with anti-infectives in morbidly obese patients undergoing abdominal surgery has been demonstrated to reduce wound infections (evidence grade A).[25,47]

Weight-based protocols were not developed for patients weighing more than 100% of ideal body weight, and there are limited data about whether total body weight, ideal body weight, or adjusted body weight correlates with the therapeutic dose.[48,49] Most heparin protocols have a ceiling weight for dosing; patients above the ceiling weight simply receive a maximum dose. Adjustment of the dose of heparin and anticoagulant in obese critically ill adults is similar to that in any critically ill adult: alter the dose based on laboratory test results. Use the activated partial thromboplastin time to dose heparin. There is no need to increase the frequency of monitoring in obese adults, but it may take longer to achieve a therapeutic goal. In addition, the absorption of subcutaneous low molecular weight heparin (LMWH) has not been well studied in the critically ill population. In healthy volunteers, a maximum dose of dalteparin (Fragmin) is recommended for patients weighing 83 kg or more, but tinzaparin (Innohep) and enoxaparin (Lovenox) do not have a cap for weight-based dosing.[50] Use serum testing of antibodies to activated coagulation factor X (anti-Xa) levels to adjust the dose and frequency of LMWH administration, especially in patients weighing more than 190 kg. Using laboratory tests to achieve therapeutic anticoagulation effects may result in new/additional costs for laboratory analysis as well as staff time and bedside resources, especially because anti-Xa factor is not routinely measured in conjunction with LMWH in the ICU.

Sedatives and opioids are lipophilic, and obese patients are at risk for drug accumulation leading to potentially prolonged effects even after ceasing administration. Opioids and sedatives are best titrated to patient response, with higher initial doses being safer when a patient has an artificial airway and is mechanically ventilated, regardless of body size. It is possible endogenous opioid concentrations may be higher in obese patients; higher endogenous opioids would result in lower-than-anticipated intravenous dosing.[51,52] One study in the perioperative setting found no differences in the amount of intraoperative sedation used in obese patients who had a BMI greater than 30 kg/m^2 and for those who had a BMI greater than 40 kg/m^2, indicating that sedation may not need adjustment to weight among obese patients in a setting that is somewhat similar to the ICU (evidence grade B).[21] Best-practice recommendations based on small, retrospective studies for pain management related to surgery in bariatric procedures (ie, weight loss surgery) include basing the dose of the opioids on lean weight.[51]

Because many drug investigation studies do not include obese or severely obese subjects, even in weight-based protocols, dosing obese critically ill patients can require additional calculations and serum analyses. For example, subjects weighing more than 109 kg were excluded in a study examining the effects of corticosteroids following acute spinal injury.[53] Methylprednisolone (Medrol) has increased clearance in extremely obese subjects compared with normal-weight patients.[54] Because of limited empiric data, it can be difficult to select the appropriate dose and administration schedule for morbidly obese patients who have traumatic spinal cord injury or other critical illnesses. Close monitoring for drug efficacy and toxicity and consultation with the clinical pharmacist are common resource-intensive interventions in the obese critically ill adult.[8,9,54,55] There are, however, limited published data describing the associations between increased monitoring or dose adjustments and outcomes such as improved glycemic control, reduced thrombotic events, or reduced toxicity in the ICU.

Consultations and Services

Most published literature includes recommendations for including a variety of health care providers in planning and implementing care of the obese patient within 24 hours of admission to the ICU.[8,9,11] Specifically, cardiac and respiratory specialists are needed to evaluate and prevent common obesity-related complications in the ICU. Morbid obesity is associated with left ventricular enlargement and dysfunction, and obese individuals are more likely to have atrial fibrillation.[56,57] Although BMI and obstructive sleep apnea are not correlated, the prevalence of sleep-disordered breathing is higher in obese patients.[58]

Additional health care providers recommended for planning and implementing care for the obese ICU patient include an APN, clinical pharmacist, physical therapist, occupational therapist, dietician, social service provider/case manager, and chaplain.[59] The APN may assist with identifying and obtaining special equipment and implementing processes that help reduce complications. Physical therapists can assist with mobility and recommend walkers or other assistive devices that meet the needs of patients according to their size. Occupational therapists can promote strength and mobility activity while the patient is in the ICU. The dietician can detail and evaluate nutritional support. Social services/case management personnel can help evaluate the discharge environment and plan for smooth transfer out of the ICU. The chaplain or another person can assist in providing psychological and emotional support as well has modeling sensitive rather than judgmental verbal communication. If the patient has a traumatic or surgical wound or skin care concerns, the wound care nurse can be consulted for optimal care. In one observational study, severely obese patients were more likely than other patients in the ICU to use additional personnel resources, regardless of their LOS.

OUTCOMES

Several unique outcomes have been reported for the obese, critically ill patient. Not all these outcomes have been found consistently in all settings. The reasons for variations in outcome are not explicit. Protocols and special training may minimize complications in the obese patient.[11,55] In one study, early involvement of the critical care clinical nurse specialist (CNS) was thought to contribute to fewer complications than anticipated in obese, critically ill patients (evidence grade B).[59] The role of the APN has great potential to contribute to safe, effective care in this population. Some of the outcomes specifically reported for obese critically ill adults are decreased mortality, LOS, wound complications, and venothromboembolism. Costs for hospital care also are an outcome of interest for this population.

Mortality

Obesity is a well-recognized comorbidity that affects both onset and recovery from illness. Obesity is recognized as an independent risk factor for increased mortality among community-dwelling adults, although the association is not consistently present among critically ill adult patients (evidence grade B).[2,5,7,60–72] Some authors suggest that it is not body size but rather other factors or comorbidities that contribute to mortality. For example, factors such as gender and increased age impact morbidity among chronically, critically ill patients.[68,70,73,74] Interestingly, in most studies comparing mortality and other outcomes of obese patients with those of normal-weight patients, obese patients often are younger and are more likely to be female, although this finding is not always statistically significant.

Wound Complications

There are conflicting data about the association between obesity and wound infection and poor wound healing. For example, several studies link obesity to impaired healing of deep and superficial sternal wounds and leg wounds after cardiac surgery (evidence grade B).[5,75] Wound complications and poorer graft survival after renal transplantation also have been associated with obesity in the hospitalized adult.[76] Obese patients undergoing major intra-abdominal surgery for cancer diagnoses have been found to have more wound complications.[77] Other studies report no increase in sternal or surgical wound healing after cardiac surgery and similar graft function after renal and liver transplant in obese patients when compared with recipients who have normal BMIs.[78–80] These differences in wound-related outcomes could result from the use of different surgical approaches or increased operating room time used when body habitus is large or could reflect altered wound dynamics when significant adipose tissue is present. Prophylactic antibiotic use in gastrointestinal surgery is supported for obese patients in the ICU (evidence grade B).[25,47]

Length of Stay

There also are conflicting data about the association of body size with LOS in critically ill patients. The relationship between obesity and LOS in the ICU and number of ventilator days has been reported as both nonexistent and positive.[2,3,7,63,64,75,81,82] LOS often was longer for severely obese patients, with a BMI greater than 40 kg/m^2, than for normal-weight patients.[2,3,70,83] Complications from infection, pulmonary embolism, wound derangements such as anastomotic leak or staple-line rupture, or the presence of multiple comorbidities requiring hourly or more frequent monitoring may require ICU admission for an obese hospitalized patient.[11,55] Because patients typically do not go directly home from the ICU, ICU admittance often results in a prolonged LOS compared with normal-weight patients who have similar surgical interventions or medical patients who have comparable comorbidities. Poor functional status and comorbidities of renal dysfunction, impaired immune status, and hypoventilation syndromes are linked to both obesity and prolonged recovery.[13,80,84–87]

Venothromboembolism

Many authors indicate that the risk for venothromboembolism (VTE) and pulmonary embolism (PE) is increased when obesity is present. In the bariatric literature, in patients undergoing gastric surgery for weight reduction, the risk of VTE does seem to be increased to 0.2% to 2.4%, compared with 1% to 2% in normal-weight hospitalized patients (evidence grade B).[88,89] Compression stockings are used to prevent VTE. A recent study suggests that proper sizing and use of compression stockings is poor in about 30% of hospitalized patients and that the sizing and application of thigh-high stockings are particularly problematic in obese patients.[90] The authors of this observational study suggest that, for VTE prophylaxis, knee-length stockings are preferable to thigh-high versions, especially for patients who have large thighs.

Costs

Increased expenses are associated with hospital care of obese patients.[91,92] Equipment to provide care for obese individuals includes bariatric gurneys, beds, wheelchairs, walkers, and bedside commodes, which must be purchased or rented (Appendix 1). Other costs include widening doorframes and installing floor-mounted commodes. Floor-mounted commodes cost about $750 and support 2000 lb, whereas wall-mounted versions supporting a maximum of 300 lb cost $350.[93] Like other structural costs, purchase or rental of bariatric equipment and costs related to renovations increase the annual medical bill of all citizens. The authors could find no estimate specific to inpatient or ICU care; one report calculated that all care for overweight and obese individuals adds an average of 37% (ie, $732) to the annual medical bill of every American.[94]

The authors could find no indication that hospitals charge more for procedures when an obese patient receives care. Rental costs for special equipment such as beds or bedside commodes generally are billed to the patient or a third-party payer. The economic advantages of renting versus purchasing have not been evaluated empirically. Anecdotal data suggest that lack of bariatric equipment may delay transfer of the obese patient from the emergency department to the ICU. Delays in transfer from the emergency department to the ICU of patients who require mechanical ventilation have been associated with increased incidence of ventilator-associated pneumonia.[92] Thus, there may be compelling reasons for purchasing equipment to avoid delays in admission or in providing optimal care caused by the process of requesting and delivering rental beds or aids to mobility.

Case Study

During the night, Ms Clark, age 49 years, is brought into the emergency department for difficulty breathing. In the emergency department it is impossible to hear any breath sounds, either normal or adventitious, and the heart sounds are extremely muffled. She has been ambulatory and independent at her apartment before admission. Her height is 67 inches; weight 249 kg (548 lbs); her BMI is 39 kg/m^2. The admission height and weight are documented, because they will be used to monitor for fluid imbalances during the hospital stay. Ms Clark has a history of type 2 diabetes mellitus, hypertension, coronary artery disease, peripheral vascular disease, and sleep apnea. At this facility, bariatric beds are rented through Purchasing. A call from the staff nurse in the emergency department initiates this process; simultaneously, the critical care APN is the ICU is alerted to the admission and alters the rental request. The APN knows that obtaining a bariatric bed with an overhead trapeze and a built-in scale as well as a lateral rotation mattress to aid in prevention of pneumonia is paramount. Other equipment needed to care for this patient, such as an extra-large blood-pressure cuff, a large wheelchair, and a bariatric-sized bedside commode, also is obtained from storage or rental companies per protocol. With timely communication, transfer from the emergency department to the ICU was not delayed. The patient is transferred to the ICU, where six staff members are needed to transfer her from the emergency department cart to the bariatric bed. The APN places an order for an air-assisted lateral transfer device that will allow safe transfers using only two personnel.

Safety issues when caring for Ms Clark are important for both the patient and the nurse. Assistance from other staff nurses and personnel will be needed for lifting, repositioning, and skin care. Some hospitals have a lift or transfer team that may be called. The critical care nurse knows that if respiratory failure occurs, intubation may be difficult because of the increased neck circumference and may take longer than usual because increased neck thickness often obstructs visualization of the larynx. Also, two people may be needed to ventilate the patient with a mask: one to hold the mask in place, and the other to manage the bagging.

The ICU nurse asks for help to reposition the patient on her left side to assess heart sounds, because this position moves the heart closer to the chest wall. Cardiac monitor electrodes are placed by locating anatomic landmarks despite the additional time it takes to do so; accurate lead placement will promote reliable ECG waveforms. The large blood-pressure cuff has a bladder that circumscribes 80% of the upper arm and does not obscure the inner elbow; a false high reading from too a small cuff is avoided. Respiratory failure is common in morbidly obese patients because fatty tissue surrounding the chest muscles leads to sleep apnea, which strains the heart, lungs, and diaphragm. The enlarged size of the chest wall and the large abdomen make lung expansion difficult. The backrest is elevated 30° to 45° using a reverse Trendelenburg position to facilitate lung expansion and prevent aspiration. Bi-level positive airway pressure (BiPAP) is ordered to help keep airways open. After three attempts to insert a peripheral intravenous line, the APN suggests a peripherally inserted central catheter (PICC) be used. Transporting the patient to radiology and back for PICC placement requires an oversized wheelchair and four personnel to position the patient on the table in special procedures. The APN notes that a project to evaluate the cost/benefit for portable equipment and staff to place PICC is needed and begins to monitor the number of PICC lines needed, the rationale for placement in ICU patients, and time from order to first use when PICC lines are placed; delay of antibiotic or other needed treatment will be noted.

In the ICU, blood glucose monitoring has been ordered four times daily, and a dietary consultation has been ordered to ensure a restricted-calorie, high-protein diet; the potential for dietary education is addressed by the dietician. During daily rounds, the critical care team includes an intensivist, bedside registered nurse, pharmacist, physical therapist, dietician, respiratory therapist, APN, and case manager; optimal interventions to avoid respiratory failure and restore health are addressed. The patient's history of peripheral vascular disease makes her prone to VTE, and peripheral automatic sequential compression stockings were placed on admission. In addition, the pharmacist discusses anticoagulation therapy, and LMWH is started with injection only into lateral thighs to attempt a more consistent absorption profile; if excess bleeding is noted, an anti-factor Xa will be added to her morning laboratory work. Morbid obesity can affect the immune system, so the nurse monitors the white blood cell count and differential and suggests adding C-reactive protein for signs of infection and/or inflammation. Physical therapy is consulted to aid with activity and mobility with the goal of maintaining independent function. The nurse encourages

Ms Clark to participate in hygiene and positioning and to perform active range of motion. She is taught to use the trapeze both for re-positioning and as a component of active range of motion. With the help of additional staff members, the nurse inspects the skin, including skin under folds, every 4 hours. The bedside nurse places a turning schedule at the bedside and helps the patient turn every 2 hours. Respiratory therapy contributes to oral hygiene and positions the patient before inhalation treatments to maximize drug distribution in the lung. Oxygen saturation is monitored closely to detect any deterioration in ventilatory status early. After 4 days in the ICU, Ms Clark no longer needs BiPAP continually, and she is transferred to a regular unit with metered-dose inhalant medications and BiPAP at night. Her bariatric bed and other equipment are transferred with her. Ongoing vigilant monitoring and interventions continue to prevent skin breakdown. The patient is discharged from the hospital 2 days later with home care as planned by the case manager.

Role of the Advance Practice Nurse

The APN is pivotal in assessing the patient, providing recommendations for specific equipment, and evaluating lifting equipment or other resources for purchase or rental by the hospital system. Both CNS and nurse practitioners manage, support, and coordinate the care of critically ill patients and can influence the optimal use of resources in the ICU. Matching the needs of the patients with staff abilities and hospital resources has the potential to reduce complications, decrease LOS, contain costs, and promote well-being.[95]

Assessment of the obese patient begins with the patient's environment. At many institutions, ordering rental equipment for care of the obese patient falls within the realm of the APN. Determining whether a special cart is needed entails more than calculation of the BMI. Generally, one should begin by determining the patient's comfort. The nurse should ask the patient directly, because what may appear to be a bed that does not provide adequate side-to-side room for moving and turning is rated by the patient as being comfortable and adequate for movement in bed. Ease of getting in and out of the bed is another aspect of the patient's bed that needs to be evaluated. Some bariatric beds do not have a low bed-to-floor profile; for obese patients who are ambulating, a bed with a high bed-to-floor profile may make getting in and out of bed awkward. In addition, a bariatric mattress often has features that promote skin health, assist with positioning, and are safer for staff. For example, the braking system on a standard bed fails at about 350 lb of force, so lifting or moving an obese patient in bed can disable brakes and may contribute to staff injury. When ordering a bariatric bed, be sure that it has a built-in scale. A trapeze for patient use in turning or moving up in bed is helpful. An air-assisted lateral transfer device may be an option associated with bed rental and should be requested to promote ease in moving or lifting the patient.

Both the CNS and the nurse practitioner can influence the care of the obese critically ill adult. The focus of the APN in the ICU is on the provision of restorative, curative, rehabilitative, palliative, and maintenance care as demonstrated by the patient's need.[96] The APN who provides care for the obese critically ill adult can minimize or prevent complications by modeling assessment techniques, anticipating and implementing care related to comorbidities, using consultation and collaboration for nutrition and drugs, and promoting teamwork in direct-care activities to prevent hazards of immobility or hypoxemia. Finally, developing technical expertise in line placement can contribute to reduced costs for both time and equipment.

When providing direct care or when teaching bedside nurses techniques for assessment, several strategies will provide accurate, reliable information. Position the obese patient to improve auscultation over adipose tissue, using a side-lying position for auscultation of posterior breath sounds. Cluster care so that each position change includes skin assessment. The APN also can plan with staff the early provision of targeted care, such as team support during turning and repositioning the obese patient.

The APN has a role in developing attitudes among nursing staff caring for obese patients. A judgmental or negative attitude can serve as a barrier to communication and cooperation among staff and contribute to dehumanizing the obese patient during the ICU stay. Intervening early and often to identify goals of care and barriers to achieving the goals are common to both the CNS and nurse practitioner roles. Addressing treatment barriers such as attitude can promote safe, effective care and reduce staff injury. Although there were no data specific to staff attitudes about obesity or care for obese patients in the ICU literature, each of the authors has heard negative comments and seen negative behaviors that do not contribute to caring practices or optimal care when the patient is obese. Self-awareness of one's own bias is one strategy to promote compassion and strategies for best practices in the care of obese individuals.

SUMMARY

Obese patients present unique challenges for daily care in the ICU setting. There is a need to identify effective assessment strategies and essential resources for optimal care and to examine the effect of interventions on outcomes and costs of care for obese hospitalized patients. An array of established and new products can assist in the care of the obese critically ill patient.

REFERENCES

1. Critical Care Statistics in the United States. 2007;1–2. Available at:http://sccmcms.sccm.org/NR/rdonlyres/1FCD55C6-71B0-48CA-B652-31EBB61DD202/504/WebStatisticsPamphletFinalJune07.pdf. Accessed November 10, 2008.
2. Tremblay A, Bandi V. Impact of body mass index on outcomes following critical care. Chest 2003;123(4):1202–7.
3. El-Solh A, Sikka P, Bozkanat E, et al. Morbid obesity in the medical ICU. Chest 2001;120(6):1989–97.
4. Pieracci FM, Barie PS, Pomp A. Critical care of the bariatric patient. Crit Care Med 2006;34(6):1796–804.
5. Ruyun J, Grunkmeir GL, Furnary AP, et al. Is obesity a risk factor for mortality in coronary artery bypass surgery? Circulation 2005;111:3359–65.
6. Lopez-Jimenez F, Malinski M, Gutt M, et al. Recognition, diagnosis and management of obesity after myocardial infarction. Int J Obes 2005;29:137–41.
7. Ray DE, Matchett SC, Baker K, et al. The effect of body mass index on patient outcomes in a medical ICU. Chest 2005;127(6):2125–31.
8. Davidson JE, Kruse MW, Cox DH, et al. Critical care of the morbidly obese. Crit Care Nurs Q 2003;26(2):105–16.
9. El-Solh AA. Clinical approach to the critically ill, morbidly obese patient. Am J Respir Crit Care Med 2004;169:557–61.
10. Marik P, Varon J. The obese patient in ICU. Chest 1998;113(2):492–8.
11. Hurst S, Blanco K, Boyle D, et al. Bariatric implications of critical care nursing. Dimens Crit Care Nurs 2004;23(2):76–83.
12. Rose DK, Cohen MM, Wigglesworth DF. Critical respiratory events in the postanesthesia care unit. Anesthesiology 1994;81:410–8.

13. Nowbar S, Burkhart K, Gonzales R, et al. Obesity-associated hypoventilation in hospitalized patients: prevalence, effects and outcome. Am J Med 2004;116:1–7.
14. Berry AM, Davidson PM, Masters J, et al. Review of oral hygiene practices for intensive care patients receiving mechanical ventilation. Am J Crit Care 2007; 16(6):552–62.
15. Bartels CL. Helping patients with dry mouth 2005:1. Available at:http://www. oralcancerfoundation.org/dental/xerostomia.htm. Published 2005. Accessed October 12, 2008.
16. Oral care in the critically ill. Practice alerts. 2007. 2. Available at: http://www.aacn. org/WD/Practice/Docs/Oral_Care_in_the_Critically_Ill.pdf. Published 2005. Accessed October 12, 2008.
17. Peerless JR, Davies A, Klein D, et al. Skin complications in the intensive care unit. Clin Chest Med 1999;20(2):453–61.
18. Solimen EZ. A simple measure to control for variations in chest electrodes placement in serial electrocardiogram recordings. J Electrocardiol 2008;41(5):395–7.
19. Drew BJ, Funk M. Practice standards for ECG monitoring in hospital settings: an executive summary and guide for implementation. Crit Care Nurs Clin North Am 2006;18(2):156–68.
20. Noninvasive blood pressure monitoring. AACN practice alert. 2006. Available at: http://www.aacn.org/WD/Practice/Docs/Noninvasive_BP_Monitoring_6-2006.pdf. Published 2006. Accessed November 12, 2008.
21. Leykin Y, Pellis T, del Mestro E, et al. Anesthetic management of morbidly obese and super-morbidly obese patients undergoing bariatric operations: hospital course and outcomes. Obes Surg 2006;16:1563–9.
22. Baugh N, Zuelzer H, Meador J, et al. Wound wise: wounds in surgical patients who are obese. Am J Nurs 2007;107(6):40–50.
23. Burns SM, Egloff MB, Ryan B, et al. Effect of body position on spontaneous respiratory rate and tidal volume in patients with obesity, abdominal distention and ascites. Am J Crit Care 1994;3(2):102–6.
24. Nelson A. Safe patient handling and movement algorithms. 2006:1–28. Available at: http://www.visn8.med.va.gov.patientsafetycenter. Published 2006. Accessed November 12, 2008.
25. Forse RA, Karam B, MacLean LD, et al. Antibiotic prophylaxis for surgery in morbidly obese patients. Surgery 1989;106:750–7.
26. Waters T, Collins J, Gainsky T, et al. NIOSH research efforts to prevent musculoskeletal disorders in the healthcare industry. Orthop Nurs 2006;25(6):380–9.
27. Brodsky JB, Lemmens HJ, Brock-Utne JG, et al. Morbid obesity and tracheal intubation. Anesth Analg 2002;94(3):732–6.
28. El Solh AA, Jaafar W. A comparative study of the complications of surgical tracheostomy in morbidly obese critically ill patients. Crit Care Med 2007;11(1):R3.
29. Heyrosa MG, Melniczek DM, Rovito P, et al. Percutaneous tracheostomy: a safe procedure in the morbidly obese. J Am Coll Surg 2006;202(4):618–22.
30. Aldawood AS, Arai YM, Haddad S. Safety of percutaneous tracheostomy in obese critically ill patients: a prospective cohort study. Anaesth Intensive Care 2008;36(1):69–73.
31. Byhahn C, Lischke V, Meininger D, et al. Peri-operative complications during percutaneous tracheostomy in obese patients. Anaesthesia 2005;60(1):12–5.
32. Kost KM. Endoscopic percutaneous dilatational tracheotomy: a prospective evaluation of 500 consecutive cases. Laryngoscope 2005;115(10 pt 2):1–30.
33. Dossett LA, Heffernaan D, Lightfoot M, et al. Obesity and pulmonary complications in critically injured adults. Chest 2008;134(5):974–80.

34. Uppot RN. The impact of obesity on radiology. Radiol Clin North Am 2007;45(2): 231–46.
35. Uppot RN, Porries W, Mueller PM. Obesity: impact on radiology. 2005. Annual Meeting. Available at: http://www.rsna.org/Publications/rsnanews/dec05/obesitydec05.cfm. Published November, 2005. Accessed November 20, 2008.
36. August D, Teitelbaum D, Albina J, et al. Guidelines for the use of parenteral and enteral nutrition in adult and pediatric patients. JPEN J Parenter Enteral Nutr 2002;26(1):S1–S138.
37. Peter JV, Moran JL, Phillips-Hughes J. A meta-analysis of early enteral versus early parenteral nutrition in hospitalized patients. Crit Care Med 2005;33(1):213–20.
38. Caba D, Ochoa JB. How many calories are necessary during critical illness. Gastrointest Endosc Clin N Am 2007;17(4):703–10.
39. Mechanick JT, Brett EM. Nutrition support of the chronically critically ill patient. Crit Care Clin 2002;18(3):587–618.
40. Stapleton RD, Jones N, Heyland DK. Feeding critically ill patients: what is the optimal amount of energy? Crit Care Med 2007;35(9):S535–40.
41. Koretz RL, Avenell A, Lipman TO, et al. Does enteral nutrition affect clinical outcome? A systematic review of the randomized trials. Am J Gastroenterol 2007;102:412–29.
42. Metheny NA. Residual volume measurement should be retained in enteral feeding protocols. Am J Crit Care 2008;72:62–4.
43. Metheny NA, Schallom L, Oliver DA, et al. Gastric residual volume and aspiration in critically ill patients receiving gastric feedings. Am J Crit Care 2008;17(6): 512–20.
44. Boullata JI. Influence of obesity on drug distribution and effect. In: Boullata JI, Armenti VA, editors. Handbook of drug-nutrient interactions. Totowa (NJ): Humana Press; 2004.
45. Erstad BL. Dosing of medications in morbidly obese patients in the intensive care unit setting. Intensive Care Med 2004;30:18–32.
46. Golan DE, Tashjihan AH, Armstrong EJ, et al. Principles of pharmacology. Philadelphia: Lippincott Williams and Wilkins; 2005.
47. Pories WJ, van Rij AM, Burlinghan BT, et al. Prophylactic cefazolin in gastric bypass surgery. Surgery 1981;90:426–32.
48. Yee WP, Norton LL. Optimal weight base for a weight-based heparin dosing protocol. Am J Health Syst Pharm 1998;55(2):159–62.
49. Spruill WJ, Wade WE, Huckaby G, et al. Achievement of anticoagulation by using a weight-based protocol for obese and nonobese patients. Am J Health Syst Pharm 2001;58(22):2143–6.
50. Phillips KW, Dobesh PP, Haines ST. Considerations in using anticoagulant therapy in special patient populations. Am J Health Syst Pharm 2008;65(15 Suppl 7): S13–21.
51. Cheymol G. Effects of obesity on pharmacokinetics: implications for drug therapy. Clin Pharm 2000;39(3):215–31.
52. Schuman R, Jones SB, Oritz VE, et al. Best practice recommendations for anesthetic perioperative care and pain management in weight loss surgery. Obes Res 2005;13(2):254–66.
53. Coleman WP, Benzel D, Cahill DW, et al. A critical appraisal of the reporting of the National Acute Spinal Cord Injury Studies (II and III) of methylprednisolone in acute spinal cord injury. J Spinal Disord 2000;13(3):185–99.
54. Blouin RA, Warren GW. Pharmacokinetic considerations in obesity. J Pharm Sci 1999;88(1):1–7.

55. Barth MM, Jensen CE. Postoperative nursing care of gastric bypass patients. Am J Crit Care 2006;15(4):378–87.

56. Wang TJ, Parise H, Levy D, et al. Obesity and the risk of new-onset atrial fibrillation. JAMA 2004;292(20):2471–7.

57. Wong CY, O'Moore-Sullivan T, Leano R, et al. Alterations of left ventricular myocardial characteristics associated with obesity. Circulation 2004;110(19):3081–7.

58. Frey WC, Pilcher J. Obstructive sleep-related breathing disorders in patients evaluated for bariatric surgery. Obes Surg 2003;13:676–83.

59. Winkelman C, Maloney B. Obese ICU patients: resource utilization and outcomes. Clin Nurs Res 2005;14(4):303–23.

60. Sjostrom LV. Mortality of severely obese subjects. Am J Clin Nutr 1992;55:516S–23S.

61. Gruberg L, Weissman NJ, Waksman R, et al. The impact of obesity on the short-term and long-term outcomes after percutaneous coronary intervention: the obesity paradox. J Am Coll Cardiol 2002;39(4):578–84.

62. Landi F, Onder G, Gambassi G, et al. Body mass index and mortality among hospitalized patients. Arch Intern Med 2000;160(17):2641–4.

63. Moulton MJ, Creswell LL, Mackay ME, et al. Obesity is not a risk factor for significant adverse outcomes after cardiac surgery. Circulation 1996;94(9 suppl):1187–92.

64. Schwann TA, Habib RH, Zacharias A, et al. Effect of body size on operative, intermediate, and long-term outcomes after coronary artery bypass operation. Ann Thorac Surg 2001;71:521–31.

65. Thompson D, Brown JB, Nichols GA, et al. Body mass index and future health-care costs: a retrospective cohort study. Obes Res 2001;9(3):210–8.

66. Smith-Choban P, Weireter LJ, Maynes C. Obesity and increased mortality in blunt trauma. J Trauma 1991;31:1253–7.

67. Troiano RP, Frongillo EA, Sobal J, et al. The relationship between body weight and mortality: a quantitative analysis of combined information from existing studies. Int J Obes Relat Metab Disord 1996;20(1):63–75.

68. Calle EE. Body-mass index and mortality in a prospective cohort of U.S. adults. N Engl J Med 1999;341(14):1097–105.

69. Bercault N, Boulain T, Keuteifan K, et al. Obesity-related excess mortality rate in an adult intensive care unit: a risk adjusted matched cohort study. Crit Care Med 2004;32(4):998–1003.

70. Goulenok C, Monchi M, Chiche JD, et al. Influence of overweight on ICU mortality: a prospective study. Chest 2004;125(4):1441–5.

71. O'Brien JM, Welsh CH, Fish RH, et al. Excess body weight is not independently associated with outcome in mechanically ventilated patients with acute lung injury. Ann Intern Med 2004;140:338–45.

72. Cawood TJ, O'Shea D, Dowd N, et al. The effect of body mass index on duration of intensive care stay and in-hospital mortality after cardiac surgery in an Irish centre [abstract]. Endocrine 2004;7:35.

73. Carson SS, Bach PB, Brzozowski L. Outcomes after long-term acute care: an analysis of 133 mechanically ventilated patients. Am J Respir Crit Care Med 1999;159:1568–73.

74. Douglas SL, Daly BJ, Brennan PF, et al. Outcomes of long-term ventilator patients: a descriptive study. Am J Crit Care 1997;6(2):99–105.

75. Potapov EV, Loebe M, Anker S, et al. Impact of body mass index on outcome in patients after coronary artery bypass grafting with and without valve surgery. Eur Heart J 2003;24:1933–41.

76. Merion RM, Twork AM, Rosenberg L, et al. Obesity and renal transplant. Surg Gynecol Obstet 1991;172(5):367–76.
77. Mullen JT, Davenport DL, Hutter MM, et al. Impact of body mass index on perioperative outcomes in patients undergoing major intra-abdominal cancer surgery. Ann Surg Oncol 2008;15(8):2164–72.
78. Hollenbeak C, Murphy D, Koenig S, et al. The clinical and economic impact of deep chest surgical site infections following coronary artery bypass graft surgery. Chest 2000;118(2):397–402.
79. Holley JL, Shapiro R, Lopatin WB, et al. Obesity as a risk factor following cadaveric renal transplantation. Transplantation 1990;49(2):387–9.
80. Engelman D, Adams DH, Byrne JG, et al. Impact of body mass index and albumin on morbidity and mortality after cardiac surgery. J Thorac Cardiovasc Surg 1999;118(5):866–73.
81. Mounsey JP, Griffith MJ, Heaviside DW, et al. Determinants of length of stay in intensive care and in hospital after coronary artery surgery. Br Heart J 1995;73: 92–8.
82. Bochicchio GV, Joshi M, Bochicchio K, et al. A time-dependent analysis of intensive care unit pneumonia in trauma patients. J Trauma 2004;56(2):296–301.
83. Yaegashi M, Jean R, Zuriqat M, et al. Outcome of morbid obesity in the intensive care unit. J Intensive Care Med 2005;20(3):147–54.
84. Kyle UG, Genton L, Pichard C. Hospital length of stay and nutritional status. Curr Opin Clin Nutr Metab Care 2005;8(4):397–402.
85. Vincent F, El-Khoury N, Rondeau E. Renal function in critically ill, morbidly ill obese patients. Respir Crit Care Med 2004;169:1332–3.
86. Berg G, Delaive K, Manfreda J, et al. The use of health-care resources in obesity-hypoventilation syndrome. Chest 2001;120(2):377–83.
87. Kessler R, Chaouat A, Schinklewitch P, et al. The obesity-hypoventilation syndrome revisited: a prospective study of 34 consecutive cases. Chest 2001; 120(2):369–76.
88. Higa KD, Boone KB, Ho T. Complications of the laparoscopic Roux-en-Y gastric bypass: 1,040 patients-what have we learned? Obes Surg 2000; 10(6):509–13.
89. Eriksson S, Backman L, Ljungstrom KG. The incidence of clinical postoperative thrombosis after gastric surgery for obesity during 16 years. Obes Surg 1997; 7(4):332–6.
90. Winslow EH, Brosz DL. Graduated compression stockings in hospitalized postoperative patients: correctness of usage and size. Am J Nurs 2008;108(9): 40–50.
91. Finkelstein EA, Ruhm CJ, Kosa KM. Economic causes and consequences of obesity. Annu Rev Public Health 2005;26:239–57.
92. Cowan MR, Trzeciak S. Clinical review: emergency department overcrowding and the potential impact on the critically ill. Crit Care Med 2005;9(3):291–5.
93. Piotorowski J, Romano M. Heavy costs: hospitals pay high price to treat obese patients [comment]. Mod Healthc 2003;33(51):10.
94. Finkelstein EA, Fiebelkorn IC, Wang G. National medical spending attributable to overweight and obesity: how much and who's paying? Health Aff 2003;(Supplement):WS219–26.
95. Maloney-Harmon PA. The synergy model: contemporary practice of the clinical nurse specialist. Crit Care Nurse 1999;22(6):101–4.
96. Bell L. Scope and standards of practice for the acute care nurse practitioner. Aliso Viejo (CA): American Association of Critical-Care Nurses; 2006.

APPENDIX 1: RESOURCES FOR CRITICALLY ILL OBESE PATIENTS

Company	Beds	Other Products
Access Medical Equipment accessmedicalequipment.com 206-365-7700	Invacare BAR600 Invacare BAR750 Invacare BAR1000	Wheelchair, commode, walker, lift chairs, scooter
Alltime Medical alltimemedical.com 866-406-3099	Invacare IVC Invacare MicroAir (mattress) Drive Medical Wt. limit 500–1000 lbs	Wheelchair, commode, walker, crutches, cane, lift chair, scooter, bed rails, footstools, overbed table, shower chair
American Medical Equipment Company medicalworldwide.com 800-394-1921	Mighty Rest Diamond Home Care Wt. limit 1000 lbs	Wheelchair, commode, walker, crutches, cane, lift, shower/transfer benches
Aria Medical Equipment ariamedical.com 800-330-3591	Invacare BAR600 Gendron 4748B-4880 Burke Tri-Flex II Camtec ExpandaCare Wt. limit 600–1000 lbs.	Lift, scales, stretchers, blood pressure cuffs, tables, footstools, chairs, physical therapy equipment
Big Boyz Industries Bigboyz.htm 1-877-574-32331-877-LRGE-BED	King's Pride 1000, King's Pride 1200 Queen's Convertible Queen's Pride 600 Wt. Limit 600–1200	—
Camtec Cambridge Tech, Inc. Camtecproducts.com. bariatricbed.html 1-800-866-1156	Bariatric Beds by Camtec Models: 4339, 4400, 4500, 4600 Wt. limit 600–1000 lbs.	Lift
ConvaQuip Ind., Inc. Convaquip.com 1-800-637-8436	Obese/Bariatric Electric Beds Wt. limit 600–1000 lbs.	Canes, lifts, mattresses, scales
CWI Medical cwimedical.com 877-9-CWIMED (1-877-929-4633)	Med Aire Plus (mattress) Wt. limit 450 lbs.	Wheelchair, commode, trapeze, lift, crutches, roller, scale, seatbelt, disposable briefs
Ergo Sciences Inc. Ergosciences.com 484-356-0211	Rehab Platform Wt. limit 600–1000 lbs.	Wheelchairs, shower/commode chair, walker, lift, stretchers
1st Senior Care 1stseniorcare.com 866-822-7348 or 877-835-8494	Drive Med Aire Whisper Lite II Eze-lok The Mighty Rest Bed Wok Diamond Homecare Wok (mattress) Tuffcare T4000F/H Tuffcare T5054HX Wt. limit 450–1000 lbs.	Wheelchair, commode, walker, lift, scale, recliner, chair

(continued on next page)

Appendix (*continued*)

Company	Beds	Other Products
Gendron Inc. Gendroninc.com 1-800-537-2521	—	Wheelchairs, commode
Hillenbrand Industries Hill-Rom.com 1-800-638-2546	Magnum II	Wheelchairs, commode, walker

Global Medical Foam
globalmedfoam.com
877-475-4260
419-884-9354
	Global care mattress
	GMF Foam mattress overlay
	(custom products
	  made based on height
	  and weight. Shipping
	  within 2 days)
		Conforming Comfort:
		Arterial heel device
		Venous stasis device
		Cervical lumbar device
		Positioning device
		Abduction device
		Wheelchair cushion
		Stretcher pads

Invacare Invacare.com/cgi-bin/ 1-800-333-6900	Invacare BAR600 Wt. limit 600 lbs.	Wheelchair, commode, walker, trapeze, cushions

KCL Kinetic Concepts Inc.
KCI1.com
1-800-275-4524
	BariAir, BariKare, BariMaxx
	  Pressure ulcer prevention
	  air loss beds
	Wt. limit 1000 lbs
		Wheelchairs, commode,
		  walker, lift, trapeze

Medical Products Direct
medicalproductsdirect.com
800-804-9549
	Invacare BAR600
	Invacare BAR750
	Tuffcare T4000
	Tuffcare T5000
	Drive
	Drive Med Aire APP
	  (mattress)
	Wt. limit 600–1000 lbs.
		Wheelchair, commode,
		  walker, lift, crutches, canes
		chair, scooter

Preferred Healthcare phc-online.com 866-553-5319	Drive #15,300-#15,303 Lumex Invacare Bar 600-1000 Titan ROHO BARISELECT (mattress) Partriot (mattress) PressureGuard (mattress) Wt. limit 600–1000 lbs.	Wheelchair, commode, walkers, transfer devices, lift chairs, trapeze, shoes, rollator (transfer device), scooter
Savion Ind. Ltd. Savion.co.il/savlinks.htm	Bariatric Care Bed Wt. limit 1100 lbs.	—
SIZEwise SIZEwise.net 1-800-814-9389	Bari-Rehab Platform, Mighty Air Wt. limit 1000 lbs.	Wheelchairs, commode, walker, lift, trapeze
Specialty Medical Supply specialtymedicalsupply.com 800-380-8539	Invacare BAR600 Invacare BAR1000 Wt. limit 600–1000	Wheelchair, commode, lift, crutches, roller
Tuffcare www.tuffcare.com	Century wide Model T4000, T5000 Wt. limit 600–1000lbs.	Wheelchairs, commode, lift, trapeze

(*continued on next page*)

Appendix (*continued*)

Company	Beds	Other Products
Universal Hospital Services uhs.com 800-847-7368	Bed frames	Wheelchair, commode, walker, lift, transfer devices, recliner, stretcher/chair
Vitality Medical vitalitymedical.com 800-397-5899	Drive Medical Bariatric Bed Drive Medical MedAire KCI BariKare bariatric bed Invacare BARPKG Wt. limit 450–4750 lbs	Wheelchair, commode, walker, crutches, rollators, lift, trapeze, scooters, transfer chair, footstool
Wheelchairs of Kansas www.WheelchairsofKansas.com/ products.lnd 1-800-537-6454	Diamond Homecare Mighty Rest Wt. limit 600–1000	Wheelchairs, commode, walker, lift

Erratum

An error occurred in the article "Continuous ST-Segment Monitoring: Raising the Bar," by Sonya A. Flanders, Volume 18, Issue 2, Page 172 (June 2006). The time measurements on page 172 in the first full paragraph and in Fig. 1 should be 0.06 seconds and 0.08 seconds.

We apologize for this oversight.

Crit Care Nurs Clin N Am 21 (2009) 423
doi:10.1016/j.ccell.2009.07.019
0899-5885/09/$ – see front matter © 2009 Elsevier Inc. All rights reserved.

ccnursing.theclinics.com

Index

Note: Page numbers of article titles are in **boldface** type.

Moving?

Make sure your subscription moves with you!

To notify us of your new address, find your **Clinics Account Number** (located on your mailing label above your name), and contact customer service at:

Email: journalscustomerservice-usa@elsevier.com

800-654-2452 (subscribers in the U.S. & Canada)
314-447-8871 (subscribers outside of the U.S. & Canada)

Fax number: 314-447-8029

Elsevier Health Sciences Division
Subscription Customer Service
3251 Riverport Lane
Maryland Heights, MO 63043

*To ensure uninterrupted delivery of your subscription, please notify us at least 4 weeks in advance of move.

Printed and bound by CPI Group (UK) Ltd, Croydon, CR0 4YY

03/10/2024

01040462-0012